PILATES

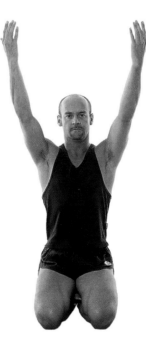

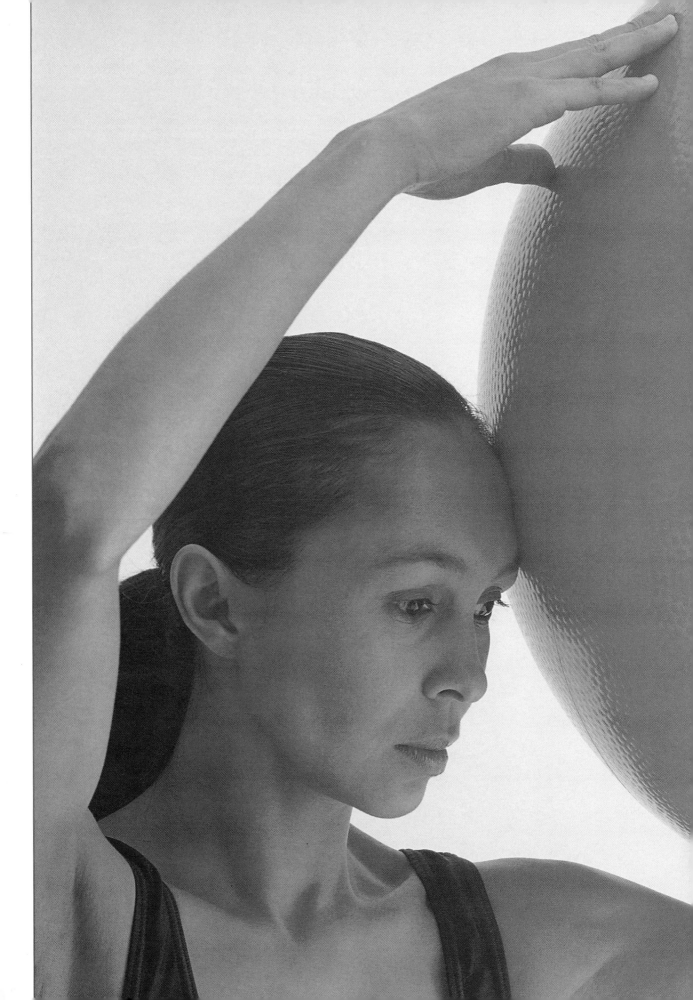

PILATES

PATRICIA LAMOND

THE LYONS PRESS
Guilford, Connecticut
An Imprint of the Globe Pequot Press

First Lyons Press edition 2002

Copyright © 2002 New Holland Publishers (UK) Ltd
Copyright © 2002 in text: Patricia Lamond
Copyright © 2002 in illustrations: New Holland Publishers (UK) Ltd
Copyright © 2002 in photographs: New Holland Image Library (NHIL)/
Ryno Reyneke, with the exception of the individual photographers
and/or their agents as listed on page 96.

First published by New Holland Publishers (UK) Ltd, 2002

ISBN 1 58574 738 6
2 4 6 8 10 9 7 5 3 1

Reproduction by Unifoto (Pty) Ltd
Printed and bound in Singapore by Craft Print (Pte) Ltd

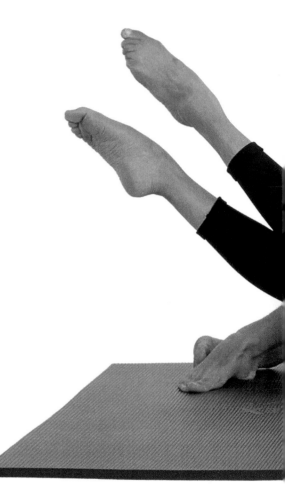

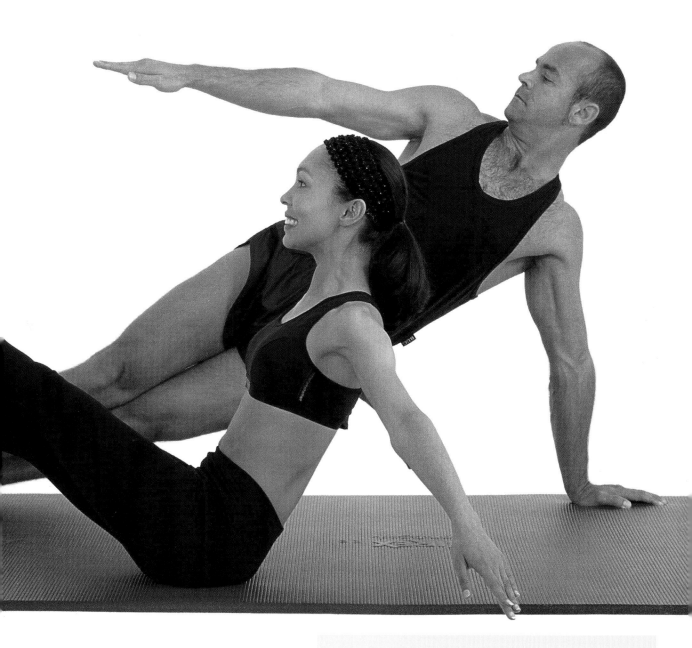

DEDICATED TO

my mother, who always achieves the impossible; and to my beloved Aub and Dal, who have always supported me in all my endeavours with unquestionable enthusiasm.

CONTENTS

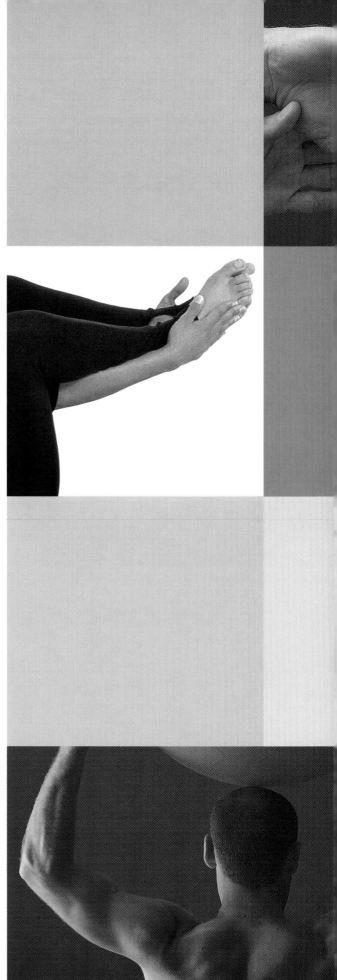

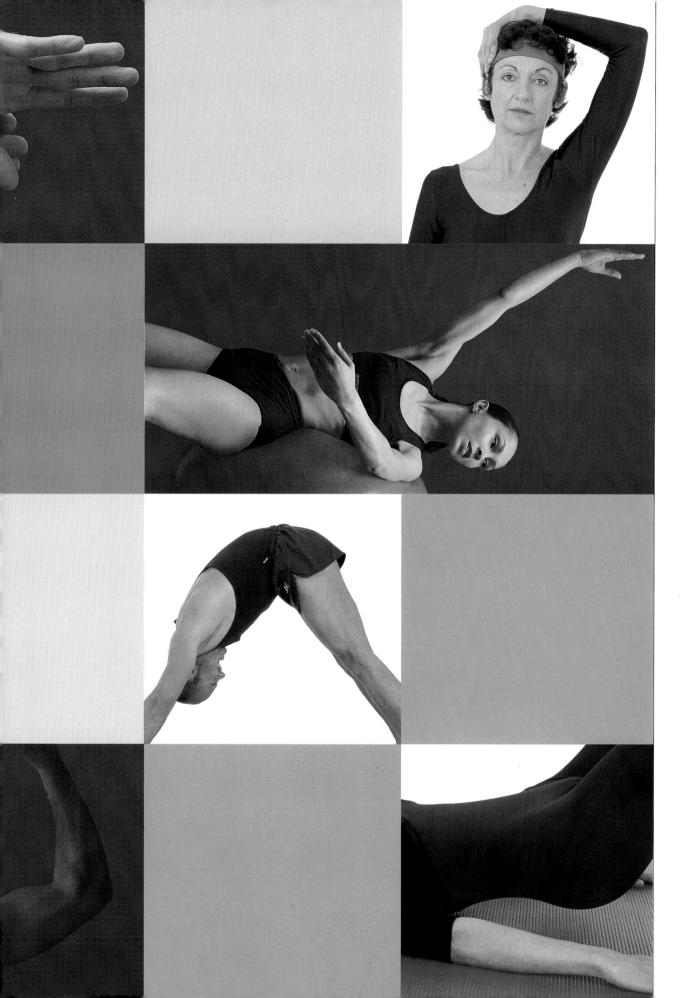

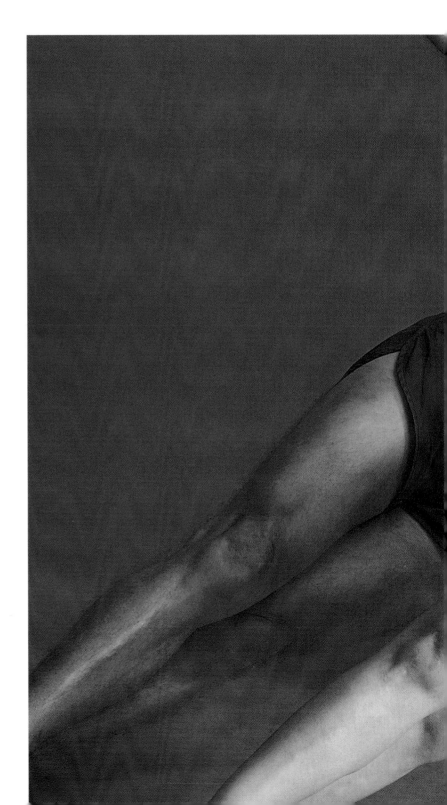

'Health is a normal
condition. It is a duty
not only to attain but
to maintain it.'

JOSEPH PILATES

'Designed to give you
suppleness, grace and skill
that will unmistakably
reflect in the way you walk,
the way you play, and the
way you work.'

JOSEPH PILATES

INTRODUCTION
TO PILATES

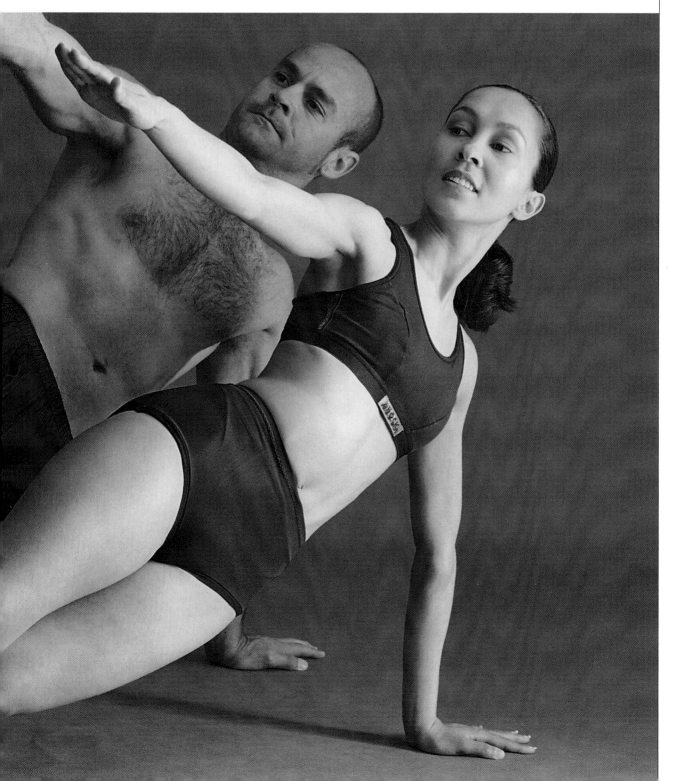

What is Pilates?

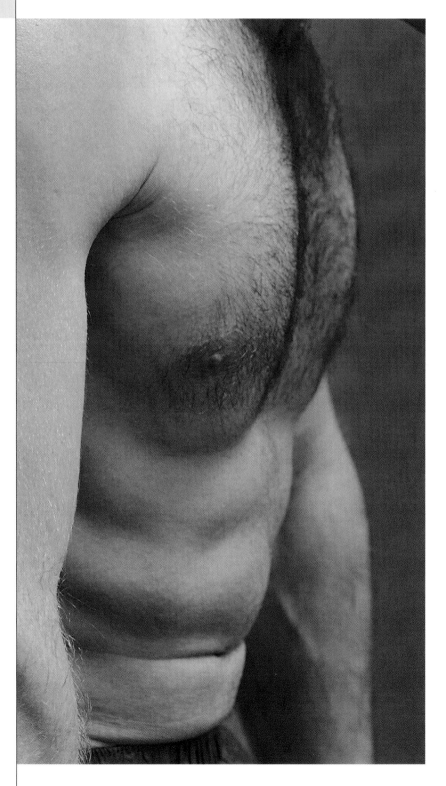

Pilates is a system of exercise developed by Joseph Pilates over 90 years ago. It is not merely another exercise fad, but a successful system that has been proved over time to achieve positive results. It is a fusion of Eastern and Western exercise in which you take control of your body, emphasizing the working of all muscles in a balanced way while remaining acutely aware of the 'mind-body' connection.

Pilates guarantees stress reduction, postural improvement, increased strength and flexibility, as well as improved tone, balance, co-ordination, circulation and overall fitness. The routine is not only for athletes, models, dancers and actors, but also for first-time exercisers, people with back problems and those in need of rehabilitative movement after injury. In addition, Power Pilates further challenges athletes who have already built up their strength.

The Pilates system of exercise targets not only the mobilizing muscles used in most exercise forms, but also the vital stabilizing muscles often neglected by other forms of exercise. A major attraction is that the exercises are varied rather than based on countless sets of repetitions. Connecting the muscles with precision and control takes focused concentration, making the smallest movement extremely powerful and challenging.

In this book you will familiarize yourself with warm-up exercises and matwork that you can do at home, in the office, or in a hotel room.

Enjoy the journey . . .

WHY PILATES?

How we treat our bodies on a daily basis influences how we feel, especially as we get older. Since much of our daily movement is unconscious, bad habits and postural misalignment can develop easily. It may be as a result of your profession, of too much sitting or sitting incorrectly, or of performing repetitive exercise that does not combine muscle balance with stretching and strengthening. The shape of your body often reflects what you do, or do not do. Pilates heightens your body awareness during your daily activities and develops the mind-body connection so that each movement becomes a conscious act controlled by the mind.

YOUR MUSCLES

The essence of Pilates is understanding where and where not to take your body. Often, people exercise muscles that are already strong, unaware of smaller, deeper muscles or how to locate them. Tense and weak muscles induced by poor posture can cause restricted, awkward and even painful movements. The harmonious muscle functioning that follows a programme of strengthening makes painless and dynamic movement possible.

Unlike other forms of exercise that work only the main muscle groups, Pilates works from the inside out, intellectualizing each muscle movement by concentrating on core stabilization from deep within the body.

Our sedentary lifestyle means we tend to develop some muscles at the expense of others, which are not used to their full potential. Through Pilates you will discover your strengths and weaknesses, and learn how to eradicate bad habits.

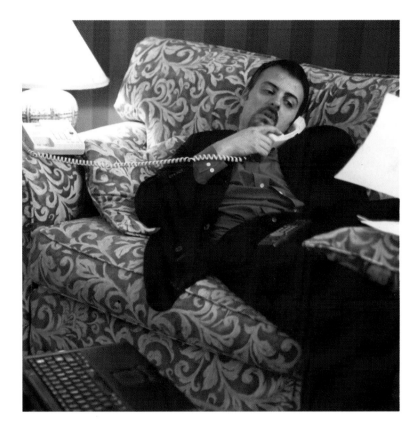

SITTING

Modern lifestyles tend to include too many hours of sitting, causing misaligned posture, which makes your body tired and tense. This can be corrected through exercise.

Once you know how, you can make a conscious effort to improve your sitting habits:
1. Feel both feet evenly placed on the floor.
2. Weight the tailbone down and centre your body.
3. Feel the tips of the ears reaching upward towards the ceiling, without tilting your head backwards.
4. Relax your shoulders and arms, and support your mid-back.
5. Lift your upper torso to create space between the hipbones and ribcage, enabling the abdominal (stomach) muscles to pull backward naturally towards the spine.
6. Take care not to push your shoulders back or extend the ribcage.

BACK PAIN

Lower back pain is one of the most common problems among adults, largely as a result of strained muscles or ligaments, or trapped spinal nerves. Pilates helps by working the deep muscles of the spine and all the abdominal muscles, creating a girdle of strength that empowers those who suffer from back pain to take charge of their problem.

Above **Slouching may appear to relax a tired back, but can compound pain and problems. Correct posture is vital.**

MENTAL AND PHYSICAL BENEFITS

'Physical fitness is the first requisite of happiness.'
JOSEPH PILATES

IN everyday life we tend to dissipate our power. Insecurities and feelings of limitation are stumbling blocks to the advancement of our being and spirit. Learning to harness your mental and physical power can improve the quality of life. Such is the power of the human mind that it can either restrict or set you free, oblivious to any limitations. Through intellectualizing the Pilates movements, you can achieve mental clarity, making the exercises more productive. The first step to intellectualizing movement is through sensory feedback and 'feeling the movement'. This accurately engages the body through the mind before you move, allowing you to exercise with accurate, uninhibited movements.

INJURY

After an injury or operation, the muscles go into protective mode, guarding the injured or painful area of the body. Many months, even years, after healing has taken place, the muscles may still be tense and weak in what was the injured area. Pain switches off the nerve fibre that connects with the muscle in the injured area. Unless retrained, the injured muscle will remain weak indefinitely. This can create an imbalance of the muscles, resulting in muscle compensation, which, in turn, places greater strain on other muscles. Sometimes, the mind believes the body is unable to return to its pre-injury state and treats the post-injury or operation area as a 'no go' area. By gradually correcting the imbalance through Pilates, the mind will more confidently accept that it is safe to exercise what was once an injured area.

TIME OUT

Our everyday lives can be noisy, rushed and cluttered – a recipe for stress, possibly even psychosomatic aches and pains. A Pilates session provides 'time out', when you take your mind inside your body, concentrating on the exercises with control, co-ordination, alignment, balance and stabilization. Centering yourself in this way requires intense concentration. To achieve physical control and co-ordination, thoughts must control actions. With controlled and continuous breathing, a sense of calm is experienced.

PHYSICAL BENEFITS

- **Fitness**
- **Stretching**
- **Muscle tone**
- **Strengthening**
- **Increased vitality**
- **Improved sex life**
- **Improved posture**
- **No more back pain**

The Pilates system is strongly underpinned by science. A single Pilates exercise or movement always includes correct postural alignment, breathing technique to engage the deeper abdominal muscles, stretching, strengthening, and accuracy of movement. Instead of the actions

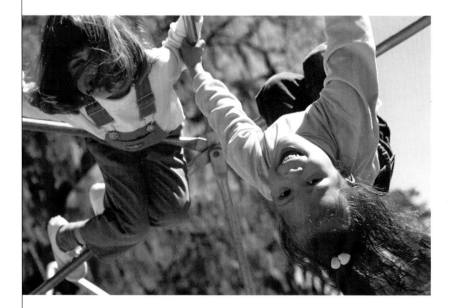

Left **Children bend, jump and tumble with great suppleness, but we tend to lose these qualitites as we mature.**

simply being choreographically correct, connections come from deep within the body, resulting in minimum movement and maximum effort, making less more. During the routine all muscles of the body are worked, starting with the deeper muscles that you cannot feel on the surface, right through to the spine. This complete fitness method improves postural awareness and develops flexibility, strength and muscle tone. Physical changes that can be achieved through Pilates are significant, such as improved posture, increased strength and a flat stomach.

RE-EDUCATION

Some people still believe in a 'no pain no gain' theory of exercise, actually associating exercise with muscle fatigue and/or soreness. By contrast, Pilates teaches that sore muscles are, in fact, the result of the build-up of waste metabolites induced by muscle imbalance, muscle fatigue through excessive repetition, torn muscles, jarring movement, and the neglect of a warm-up and stretching programme.

The Pilates method includes anatomical awareness, which, combined with consciousness for full mind-body awareness, should leave you feeling neither mentally nor physically exhausted.

Pilates has long been practised by famous people such as dancer Martha Graham, actors Gregory Peck, Audrey Hepburn and Jodie Foster, tennis star Pat Cash and rock icon Madonna. International rugby and cricket teams all over the world are including Pilates in their training programmes in order to reduce the risk of injuries.

JOSEPH PILATES
Man and mentor 1880–1967

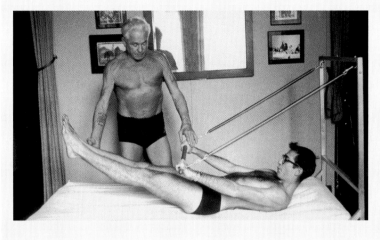

Joseph Humbertus Pilates was born in Germany, a sickly child who suffered from asthma, rheumatic fever and rickets. Determined to conquer his debilities and improve his physical condition, he went on to become an accomplished gymnast, skier, boxer, body builder, competitive swimmer and self-defence trainer.

Taking a keen interest in karate and yoga, he combined Eastern and Western exercise disciplines to establish the mind–body concept that lies at the heart of the Pilates system. Ancient Greek philosophy also served as an inspiration.

Interned in a prisoner of war camp during World War I, Pilates helped guards and prisoners to maintain fitness. Using his bunk, bedsprings and chair, he improvised the creation of the apparatus that was to become the Reformer, Trapezium (pictured above) and Wunda chair still found in Pilates studios today. During this period, a devastating influenza epidemic spread across the globe, claiming 50 million lives. Miraculously, there were no influenza casualties in Pilates' camp, a fact attributed directly to the fitness of the men. The British army then employed Pilates to assist in training the British troops. After the war, he emigrated to the United States where he and his wife, Clara, set up the first Pilates studio in New York in 1926.

The famous Russian choreographer, George Ballanchine of the New York City Ballet, was soon sending his dancers to Pilates' classes. The dance pieces known as the 'Seven Deadly Sins', choreographed by Ballanchine, incorporate the Pilates mat routine. American, Martha Graham, doyenne of 20th century modern dance, also studied with Pilates, drawing on his movements in the development of the Graham technique.

Pilates passed away at the age of 87 in 1967, but left a powerful legacy that will continue to benefit many people for years to come.

CHOOSING A PILATES TEACHER

A Pilates book or video serves as a guide and is useful to reinforce knowledge you may already have gained on the subject. However, the finer points, as well as the mental and physical depth of the subject, may be missed or misconstrued if it is your only teacher.

It is always advisable to consult a Pilates instructor to check that your placement is correct. A good Pilates teacher will also be able to advise you on your personal strengths and weaknesses, and to devise a programme specifically suited to your ability and requirements. With guidance, you will progress steadily to reach your full potential.

The full Pilates programme consists of both matwork and equipment-based exercises. An equipped Pilates studio will have a Reformer, Trapezium (also known as a Trap table or Cadillac), Wunda chair, various barrels, physio balls of different sizes, thera-bands and fitness circles. On the machines, you will work against resistance and become acutely aware of exactly what each particular exercise is emphasizing and expecting from your body. This will enable you to understand depth and control of movement more clearly. What you learn on the machines will apply to your matwork, too, helping to make it even more effective.

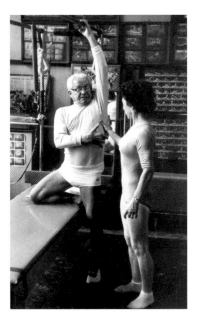

Above **Joseph Pilates demonstrates a movement on the Trap table, also known as the Trapezium or Cadillac.** *Left* **A Pilates teacher can help you to build the balance, strength and control needed to achieve ease of movement in this side bend exercise.**

With individual tuition you will learn from the beginning to do the exercises properly. Under the teacher's watchful eye, you will engage the body accurately and target the appropriate muscles for each specific exercise.

Many health and fitness trainers are incorporating Pilates into their work, often without sufficient knowledge of either anatomy or the mental and physical depth of Pilates.

The importance of the applied Pilates principles in the exercises cannot be overemphasized. Risk of injury is increased if the principles regarding placement (neutral spine, ribcage, scapular and shoulder girdle placement) and stabilization are not maintained.

It is imperative to choose an experienced, reputable teacher who has attained accredited certification from a recognized Pilates institution.

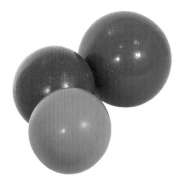

Physio balls

The barrel

Professional reformer

Split and raised floor mats

Above **Pilates equipment was originally developed by German gymnast and body builder, Joseph Pilates. Today's equipment is sophisticated and well-engineered.**

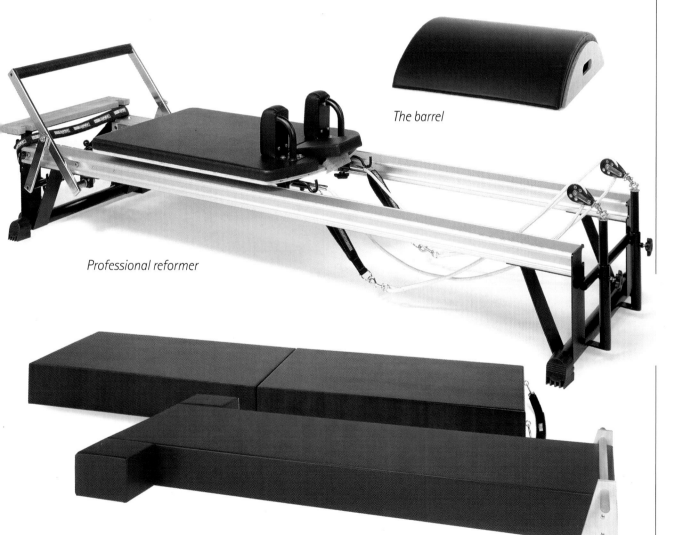

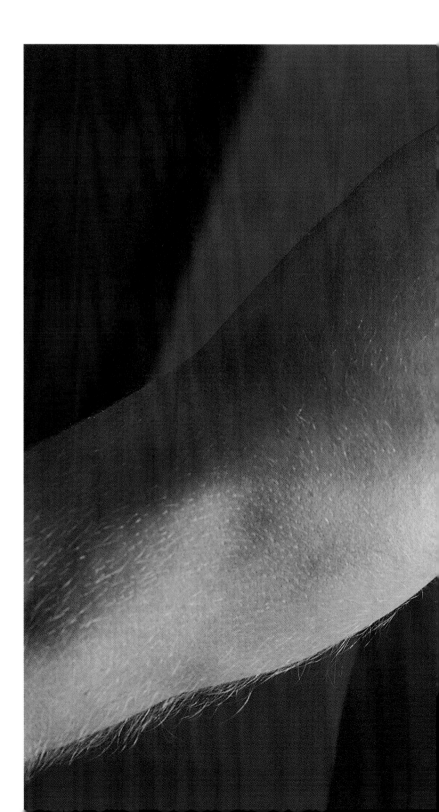

'Pilates develops the body uniformly, corrects wrong postures, restores physical vitality, invigorates the mind and elevates the spirit.'

JOSEPH PILATES

'A man is only as young as his spinal column.'

JOSEPH PILATES

UNDERSTANDING YOUR BODY

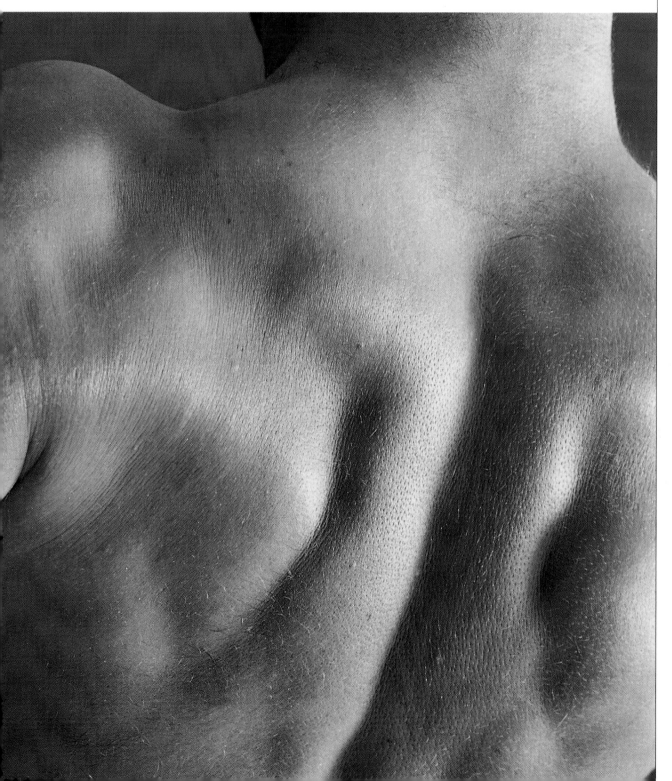

ANATOMY

*'Each muscle may co-operatively and loyally aid
in the uniform development of all our muscles.'*

JOSEPH PILATES

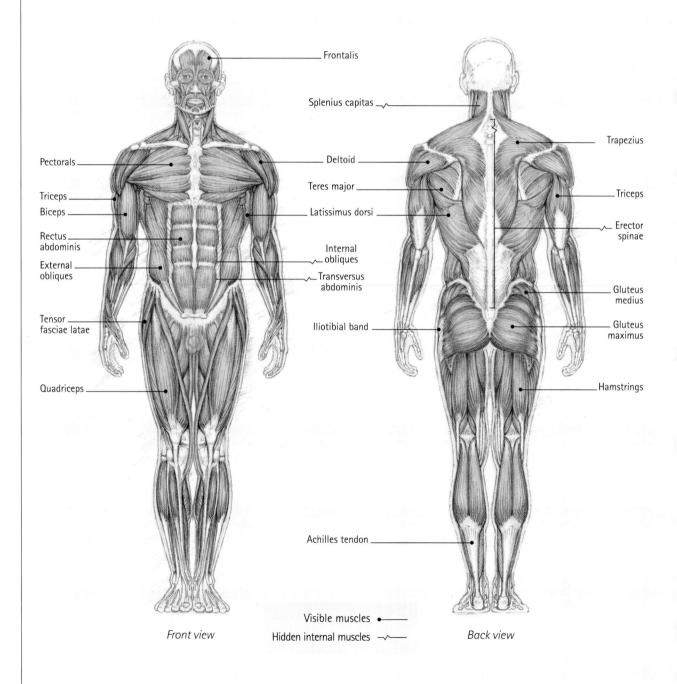

Frontalis

Splenius capitas

Trapezius

Pectorals

Deltoid

Teres major

Triceps

Triceps

Biceps

Latissimus dorsi

Erector
spine

Rectus
abdominis

Internal
obliques

External
obliques

Transversus
abdominis

Gluteus
medius

Tensor
fasciae latae

Iliotibial band

Gluteus
maximus

Quadriceps

Hamstrings

Achilles tendon

Visible muscles ●———

Hidden internal muscles ✓———

Front view

Back view

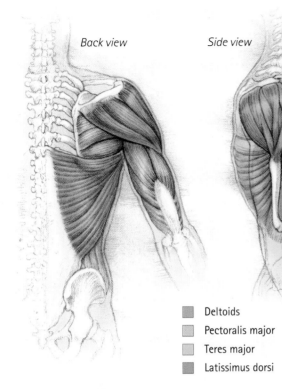

Back view   *Side view*

- Deltoids
- Pectoralis major
- Teres major
- Latissimus dorsi

THE neuromuscular or mind-body connection of Pilates makes it vital for practitioners to gain a basic understanding of anatomy, especially the muscular-skeletal section.

The precision with which the Pilates movements are executed requires acute awareness of the muscles selected for an exercise, even before taking those muscles into motion.

Carefully study the illustrations in this section to improve your knowledge and enhance your workout.

Splenius muscles

Action: Movement of the head and neck into cervical extension (looking up), rotation and turning the head to the side.

Application: The splenius muscles bring the upper trapezius and Erector spinae into play.

Deltoid muscles

Action: Applied in arm lifting movements.

Application: The trapezius stabilizes the scapula and the deltoid pulls on the humerus (upper arm) during arm lifting.

Trapezius muscles

Upper trapezius

Action: Elevation of the scapulae (lifting the shoulder blades) and extension of the head (looking up).

Mid trapezius

Action: Elevation of the scapula and adduction (pulling shoulder blades together).

Lower trapezius

Action: The lower trapezius pulls shoulder blades down and enables circular lifting movements of the scapulae.

Application: When all parts of the trapezius work together, they pull upward and push the shoulder blades together at the same time. When you lift an object overhead, the trapezius holds the shoulder blades against the ribcage.

Latissimus dorsi

Action: Pulls the entire shoulder girdle down.

Application: Felt in all exercises pulling the arms down.

Pectoralis major

Action: Aids the Latissimus dorsi, e.g. a gymnast working in rings, where the arms are lengthened and kept close to the body.

Application: Used in push-ups, pull-ups, throwing, stretching the arm.

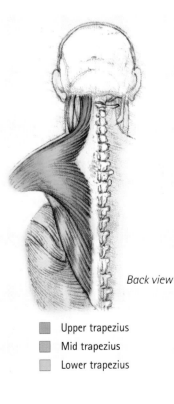

Back view

- Upper trapezius
- Mid trapezius
- Lower trapezius

Back view   *Side view*   *Side view*   *Side view*   *Front view*

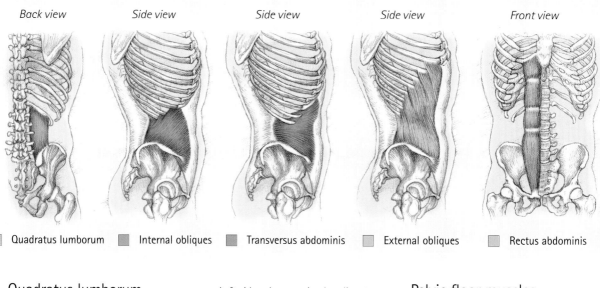

☐ Quadratus lumborum   ■ Internal obliques   ■ Transversus abdominis   ☐ External obliques   ■ Rectus abdominis

Quadratus lumborum

Action: Stabilizes the pelvis and the lumbar (lower spine) area.
Application: Applied in lumbar extension (when lower spine arches backward) and lumbar lateral flexion (lower spine bending sideways).

Rectus abdominis

Action: Spinal lumbar flexion (lower spine bending forward).
Application: Spinal flexion.

Transversus abdominis

Action: Forced expiration (breathing out), pulling abdominal wall inward.
Application: This is the main muscle of forced expiration, assisted by the Rectus abdominis and the external and internal obliques. It is the main 'corset' muscle that holds the abdomen flat.

External oblique

Action: Both sides – lumbar flexion (lower spine bending forward).

Right side – lower spine bending to the right, or lower spine turning to the left.

Left side – lower spine bending to the left, or lower spine turning to the right.
Application: These muscles on either side of the trunk can work independently. Working together, they aid the Rectus abdominis, for example, in flexing the spine when getting out of bed. Each side of the external oblique must be stretched individually.

Internal oblique

Action: Both sides – lumbar flexion (lower spine bending forward). Right side – lower spine bending sideways to the right or turning to the right. Left side – lower spine bending sideways to the left or turning to the left.
Application: The muscle fibres of the internal obliques run diagonally in the opposite direction to those of the external obliques. The left internal oblique rotates the torso to the left and the right internal oblique rotates the torso to the right. In turning movements, the internal oblique and external oblique on opposite sides work together.

Pelvic floor muscles

Action: Compresses the abdomen, is active in forced expiration (breathing out), contracts the vaginal muscles in women, and the urethra in men.
Application: Contraction while urinating is an example of how to apply this muscle.

Quadriceps

This consists of four muscles: Rectus femoris, Vastis lateralis, Vastis intermedius and Vastis medialis.
Action: All four muscles attach to the kneecap and are knee extensors. Rectus femoris assists in hip flexion.
Application: The quadriceps act as decelerators to decrease speed or change direction. People with good jumping ability have strong quadriceps.

Iliopsoas

This consists of the iliacus, Psoas major and Psoas minor.
Action: Bending at the hip, and turning the legs outwards.
Application: Activated when raising the legs from the floor while lying on your back.

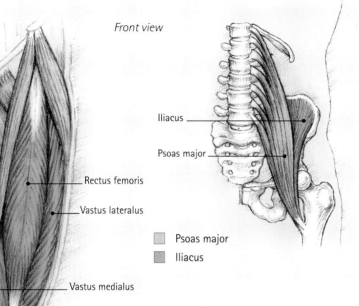

Front view

Iliacus

Psoas major

Rectus femoris

Vastus lateralus

Vastus medialus

Quadriceps

Psoas major

Iliacus

BACK PROBLEMS

The Psoas major tends to move the lower back forwards. In a supine position, it pulls the back up as it raises the legs – and can possibly aggravate lower back problems. Very low leg raises are not recommended for those with back problems. The abdominal muscles prevent the weight of the legs from pulling the pelvis forward and arching the back, helping to prevent lower back pain.

Gluteus maximus

Action: Hip rotation and extension. Lower fibres assist in adduction (medial movement towards the midline of the trunk).

Application: Running, hopping, skipping, jumping and returning from a squatting to a standing position.

Gluteus medius

Action: Hip rotation.

Application: In walking, when the body is balanced on one leg, they prevent the opposite hip from sagging.

Gluteus minimus

Action: Abduction of the hip (lateral movement away from the midline of the trunk). Internal rotation as the femur abducts.

Application: Both Gluteus minimus and Gluteus medius are used in running, hopping and skipping, where the body weight is passed from one foot to another.

Tensor fasciae latae

Action: Rotates the hip internally as it flexes; abduction of the hip (e.g. raising the upper leg when lying on your side); and forward bending from the hip.

Application: This muscle helps to prevent external rotation. It is used when you unconsciously turn the foot inwards when walking or running, which is a weak position. Lying on your back and raising the leg with the femur turned inwards will also activate it.

It may be developed in side-lying positions, lifting the leg and slowly lowering it back to rest against the other leg.

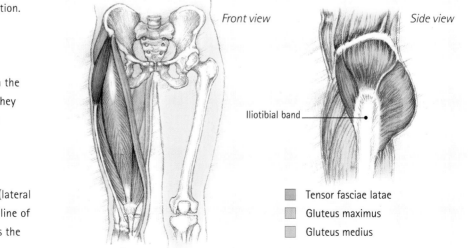

Front view

Side view

Iliotibial band

Tensor fasciae latae

Gluteus maximus

Gluteus medius

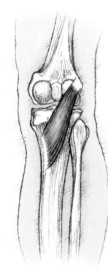

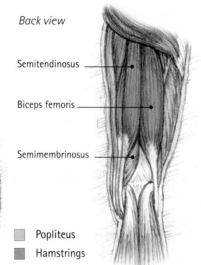

Back view

Semitendinosus

Biceps femoris

Semimembrinosus

Popliteus
Hamstrings

Erector spinae

Action: Extension and sideways bending of the spine.

Application: The largest muscle in the spinal column, it keeps the body upright. It functions when the pelvis is neutral (tilting neither backwards nor forwards), and the spine is lengthened. Strengthening exercises are usually performed lying on the stomach.

Multifidi

Action: Extension and contra-lateral rotation (opposite side twisting) of the spine.

Application: These deep spinal muscles are responsible for stabilizing each vertebra on top of the next. When the Transversus abdominis is engaged (using Pilates' 'belly to spine' technique) the multifidi stabilize the lumbar area.

Hamstrings

These antagonists (opposing muscles) to the quadriceps, are situated at the back of the thigh, and are responsible for knee bending. They consist of three muscles:

1. Biceps femoris
Action: Knee bending, turning the knee outwards, and hip extension (lengthening muscles at the back of the leg).
2. Semitendinosus
3. Semimembrinosus
Action: Semitendinosus and Semimembrinosus, assisted by the popliteus muscle behind the knee, are responsible for knee bending and turning it inwards.
Application: The hamstrings are often referred to as the 'running muscles' because of their accelerating function. Hamstring strain is common in sports requiring explosive running.

Special exercises to improve hamstring strength and flexibility are important.

Popliteus

Action: Assists the hamstrings in unlocking the knee to bend.

Application: This muscle is the only true flexor of the leg at the knee and is vital for knee stability. It assists the hamstrings and is used in walking and running.

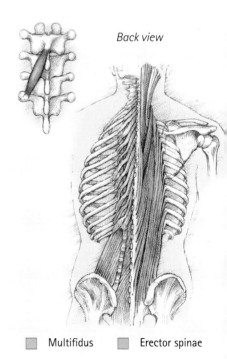

Back view

Multifidus   Erector spinae

POSTURAL ALIGNMENT

POSTURAL analysis will help you to understand your body before you embark on a Pilates exercise routine for the first time. Anyone over 40 years old should also have a pre-exercise medical check-up, especially when exercise has not previously been a priority. As with any exercise programme, pregnant women and anyone being treated for specific medical conditions, such as heart disease or blood pressure, should consult a doctor before embarking on the Pilates programme.

POSTURAL ANALYSIS

Although many people look at themselves in a mirror without really seeing their own postural imbalances, identifying them is crucial. Only by addressing the imbalances of the muscles and the incorrect movement patterns that have evolved over time can Pilates bring the body back to its balanced state.

Look at the illustrations of misplaced posture and/or muscle imbalances on this page and pages 28–30. Do you recognize yourself in one or more of them? Once you have identified your own postural deviations, start working on correcting your alignment or muscle imbalance.

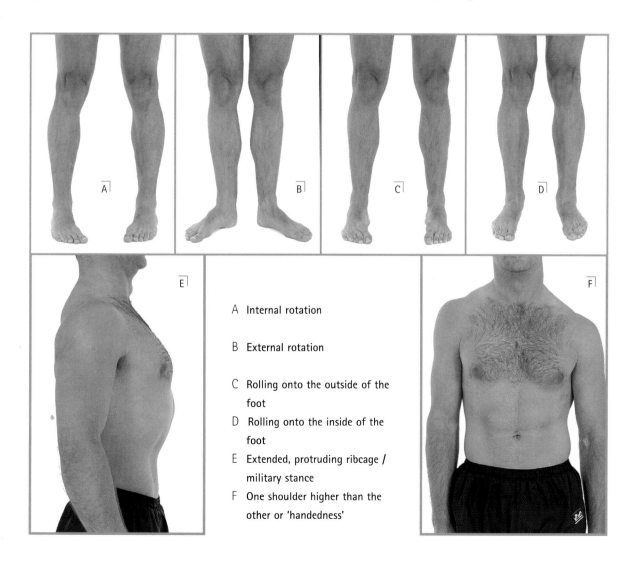

A Internal rotation

B External rotation

C Rolling onto the outside of the foot

D Rolling onto the inside of the foot

E Extended, protruding ribcage / military stance

F One shoulder higher than the other or 'handedness'

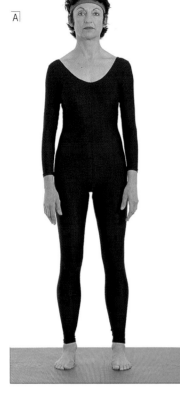

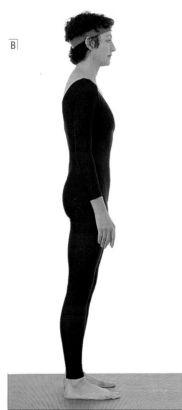

CORRECTING AND IMPROVING POSTURE

1. **Legs:** Stand in front of a full-length mirror, legs hip-width apart, feet parallel, thigh muscles engaged, knees extended but not hyper-extended (i.e. do not push into the back of the knees).

2. **Feet:** Aim to align the kneecap with the centre of the foot, and balance the weight of the body evenly over both feet, avoiding inward or outward rolling of the feet.

3. **Neutral pelvis:** Place your fingers on the hipbones and align both hipbones with the pubic bone so that all three are on the same plane. There should be neither a forward nor backward pelvic tilt.

4. **Torso:** Imagine gently pulling the bottom ribs in and slightly down towards the hipbones. Now lift the breastbone without disturbing the ribcage placement.

5. **Head and shoulders:** Engage the lower trapezius and slide the shoulder blades down towards the hips. Retain equal shoulder placement, without one shoulder being higher than the other. Balance the head perfectly on top of the spine without tilting it to one side, and position the forehead slightly in front of the chin to avoid shortening the back of the neck.

Top left **Frontal view showing correcting postural alignment, with neutral pelvis and knee directly over the centre of the foot.**
Left **Side view showing head too far forward. The ear should be above the shoulder for correct alignment.**

STABILIZING AND MOBILIZING MUSCLES

The Pilates system of exercise emphasizes the role of the stabilizing muscles. Stabilizers are muscles that surround a joint or body part, stabilizing it by holding the bones in place and allowing another limb or body part to move. Mobilizing muscles are responsible for larger movements. Ideally, the mobilizers should mobilize and the stabilizers should stabilize. Stabilizing muscles start to lose their effectiveness when they begin to act more as mobilizing muscles. A good example is when you do sit-ups without any knowledge of how to engage the stabilizers. For sit-ups to be effective, the Transversus abdominis and obliques should be consciously engaged. When they are not, they become movers (mobilizers).

During everyday activities, the lower spine and pelvic area are not usually stabilized. The reason Pilates is effective for people with back problems is because it concentrates on strengthening the stabilizing muscles supporting the spine.

SYNERGIST MUSCLES

These muscles assist in refined movement and rule out undesired movement.

BODY-ALIGNMENT AND THE JOINTS

The muscles support the body in its natural state when the body is accurately aligned. If the relationship of the joints is not correct when you exercise, undue stress and muscle imbalance is the result. Conscious, correct alignment should therefore precede all exercise movements.

There are many types of joints. Some are immovable, others are slightly movable, whilst the freely movable joints are known as the synovial joints. Covered with cartilage, they are lubricated by synovial fluid. Without lubrication, osteoarthritis may develop. Movement and exercise lubricate the cartilage surrounding the joints. All joints affect one another. If, for example, the hip is a problem area, pain may be manifested in the knee – a phenomenon known as referred pain. When the hip is correctly aligned, however, the knee pain disappears.

AGEING AND THE SPINE

As we age, it often becomes apparent that one side of the body is more developed than the other, because the balance is not maintained between the muscles in front of the spine and those behind it. This can cause pain and discomfort.

With too much sitting, the abdominal muscles become weaker. This, in turn, induces weak back muscles and poor posture. To stay upright the Erector spinae have to overwork, becoming tight and strong, whereas the abdominals become lengthened and weak.

Excessive repetitions of forward, back or side bending movements will impair the balance and pressurize the discs of the spine. Most people do not have a straight spine. Although some disorders, such as scoliosis and kyphosis, may not be easy to correct, working to strengthen the muscles will help to lessen the strain that could develop into pain.

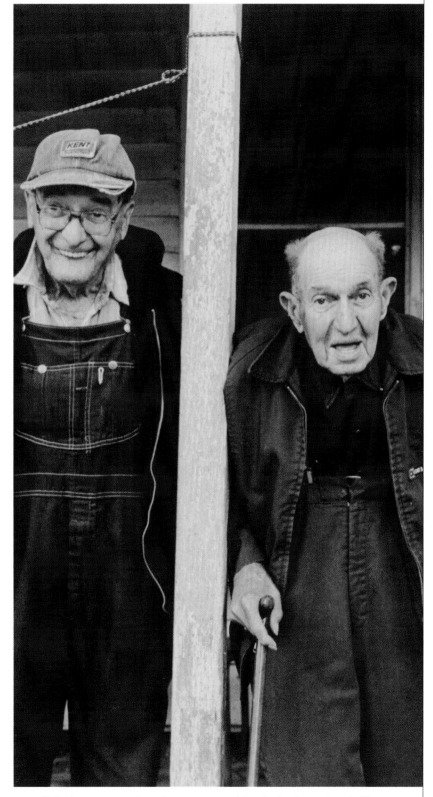

Above **Believing a man to be only as young as his spinal column, Joseph Pilates advocated strengthening and balancing exercises to reduce strain.**

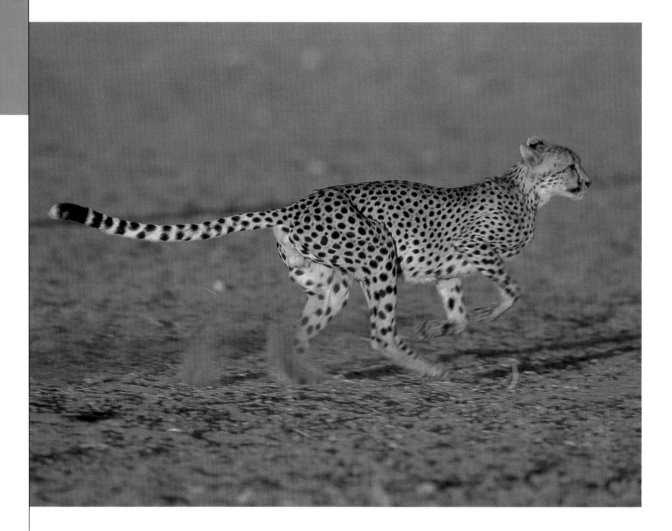

ANIMAL MOVEMENT

Humans tend to focus on one area alone instead of utilizing all the muscles, whether they are sitting, standing, walking or running. An animal stretches from head to toe when it moves from a supine to a standing position.

Animals have a natural suppleness, balance, strength and vitality. Joseph Pilates believed that human movement should be as natural as animal movement. Some Pilates exercises are even named after animals, for example, 'the swan', 'the seal' and 'cat stretch'.

LIFESTYLE, MOVEMENT AND SPORT

Newborn babies and young children do not have muscle imbalances or poor posture. Indeed, much poor posture has to do with Western lifestyle. Muscular-skeletal imbalance can be induced by many things, such as your type of employment, workstation (e.g. desk or kitchen counter), chairs providing inadequate support, daily tasks,

Above **Pilates believed humans should strive to emulate the natural, supple grace of animal movement.**

illness, injury, stress, sport, and lack of postural awareness. To a certain extent, too, posture may be hereditary. Whatever the cause, it should be addressed and improved.

Muscle imbalance occurs when certain muscles are lengthened (often due to poor posture) whilst others are shortened – for example, when a person sits hunched forward over a desk. In this hunched position the upper trapezius muscle takes over. The upper trapezius and the pectoral muscles are shortened, while the lower trapezius muscle is lengthened and gets weaker. The Lattisimus dorsi

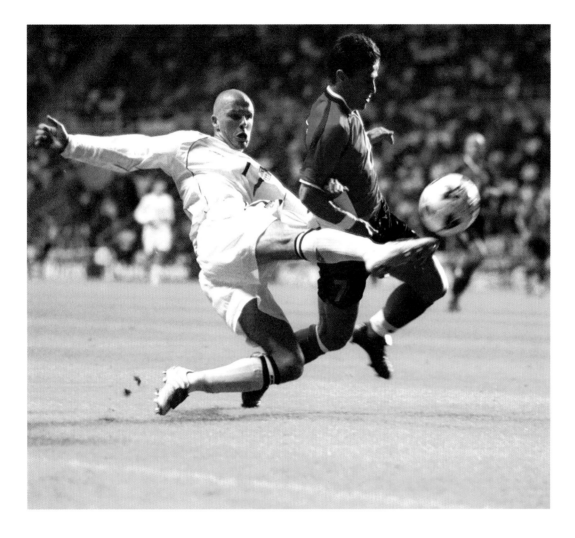

and the lower trapezius should work as stabilizers to keep the shoulders pulled down correctly. If not, the imbalance causes the larger muscles in the body to compensate, taking over the movement and causing ineffective movement patterns that evolve into bad habits through repetition.

Sport creates specific repetitive movement, adding to the body's muscle imbalance. Most fitness regimes hone in only on the mobilizing muscles. Problems arise when the mobilizing muscles act as stabilizers because the stabilizers become inactive. Where shortened muscles do not contract

properly, they cannot release the opposing muscles correctly. Muscle imbalance and inaccurate movement are the result.

Ideal posture is achieved through balanced action, which occurs when the stabilizing muscles are not only fully activated but assist the mobilizing muscles. The body is then supported in a natural, unstressed way with correct muscle synergy.

Above **Pilates can help sportsmen to reduce muscle stress arising from repetitive movement.**

UNDERSTANDING YOUR OWN BODY

Most people have muscle imbalances, which can develop into physical problems. Pilates movements require a cerebral approach and an understanding of your own body. Once misaligned posture has been corrected or improved, the body can be strengthened through Pilates movements. By exercising specific muscles, correct movement patterns are re-established.

Your body is your responsibility. Take charge of it and take charge of your life. All you have to do is put your mind to it.

WORK ON THE WEAK AREAS

WORKING on the weak areas means re-educating your muscles. When muscles and ligaments do not offer the correct support, the joints exceed their normal range, pulling on the ligaments and joint capsules. This results in faulty alignment or bad posture, leading to undue stress and strain on bones, joints and muscles.

Everyone is different, so take care to analyze and understand your own postural imbalances. Then invest time and effort to correct the weak areas of your body.

OVERLOADING THE MUSCLES

The basic principle of exercise is overloading the muscles, which become stronger in response to the load placed on them. However, unconscious strengthening through overloading the muscles will not always deliver results over a short period. Without knowledge of the body's anatomy and an understanding of your own strengths and weaknesses, you may not achieve a marked increase in muscle tissue or strength. If, however, you exercise consciously, with clear objectives, applying less load over a longer period, more positive results are likely to be achieved.

Overloading is not always a natural progression in exercise. In some cases, the load should be reduced to achieve the desired results. Frequency, intensity and duration should always be considered. When muscles become fatigued, other mus-

cles are called upon to assist in the exercise – defeating the object of exercising specific muscles or groups of muscles. More importantly, injury looms if muscles are tired.

SPECIFIC ADAPTATIONS TO IMPOSED DEMANDS

Over time, the body adapts and accepts stresses to which it is constantly subjected. Conscious adaptation to correct posture, as well as knowledge of the muscles and skeletal alignment, will enable you to strengthen weak areas using specific muscles for the movements for which they are intended. Understanding how to employ specific muscles for a specific exercise is a Pilates pre-requisite.

BE SPECIFIC

Strength, endurance and flexibility vary from one group of muscles to another, as well as from one individual to another. A specific exercise may not be appropriate for your individual requirements. Body composition must

be taken into account regarding repetitions and weight training. Working on equipment not suitably adjusted to your height, strength or ability is unintelligent exercise.

HANDEDNESS PATTERNS

'Handedness' is a condition in which one shoulder is higher than the other, and it is typical where one side of the body is dominant. The body of a right-handed person may become more developed on the right side. Usually, there is a slight deviation of the spine, with one hip higher than the other. Standing in front of a mirror and tilting the pelvis sideways to level the hips will temporarily correct the imbalance. What is more difficult, however, is to maintain the correct balance at a conscious level. ncreasing the repetitions of an exercise on the weaker side of the body, combined with correct body alignment, helps to balance handedness patterns.

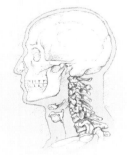 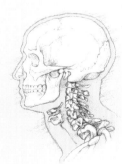

Above left **Correct alignment of the cervical spine.** *Above right* **Extension of cervical spine, with rounded upper back and chin 'jutting' forward (poking chin).**

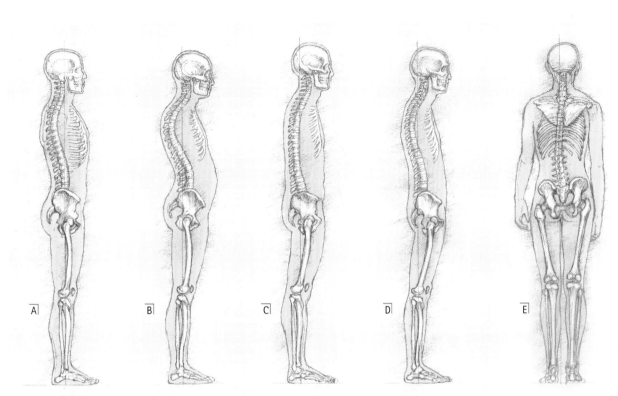

PROTRACTION OF THE HEAD (CHIN 'JUTTING' FORWARD)

The pattern in which the skull moves forward and the chin 'juts' out is accompanied by an increased cervical lordosis (hollow back). When the upper back slumps, there is a compensatory change in the position of the head and neck. Good upper back alignment is needed to restore correct head and neck alignment so as not to strain muscles.

To correct head alignment:

1. Open the pectorals, pull the mid-back downwards and engage the Latissimus dorsi.

2. Increase the length between the bottom of the skull and the neck and feel the tips of the ears pulling upwards. Feel the back of the neck lengthen. Imagine your head perfectly balanced on top of a skewer.

A **Ideal alignment**
B **Kyphosis-lordosis posture**
C **Flat-back posture**
D **Sway-back posture**
E **Scoliosis posture**

UPPER BACK AND NECK TENSION

When the upper body is correctly positioned, the spine is erect without exhibiting an exaggerated cervical ordosis or kyphosis.

Scapular stabilization helps to alleviate neck and upper body tension. Engaging the lower trapezius and shoulder girdle muscles provides stability to the scapulae, serving as a support base for shoulder activity. Opening the pectorals and pulling down the Latissimus dorsi towards the waist aids scapular stability.

Adequate strengthening of the rotator cuff muscles will provide endurance and ensure proper functioning.

KYPHOSIS

The spine between the shoulder blades is normally convex to the back. However, it is abnormal if it becomes a hump-like curvature. Even though the lower back may be strong, the upper back, Erector spinae and neck flexors may be weak. Habitual positions and activities often give rise to the development of a lordosis-kyphosis posture, where the one compensates for the other, and may be thecause of substantial muscular-skeletal imbalance. Kyphosis is associated with osteoporosis. The kyphotic posture should not be confused with round shoulders, although in fact the one might accompany the other in some cases.

Opening the pectorals, pulling the mid-back downwards and engaging the Lattisimus dorsi will help to improve kyphosis.

MUSCLE IMBALANCE

This is an imbalance of strength between the agonist and antagonist, for instance, strong quadriceps (agonist) and weak hamstrings (antagonist).

Muscles that are shortened tend to be stronger than their antagonist muscles, whereas muscles that are lengthened tend to be weaker than their antagonist muscles. An example of this is where the upper trapezius and pectorals are stronger and tighter and the lower trapezius and Lattisimus dorsi are weaker. This results in a hunched upper body posture which could be the result of sitting behind a desk without postural awareness.

THE SHOULDER JOINT AND SHOULDER GIRDLE

The position of the arm and shoulder joint depends on the position of the scapula. In ideal alignment, the scapulae lie flat against the back. Faulty positioning of the scapulae has the negative effect of misaligning the shoulder joints.

Pilates exercises performed in the prone position (on your stomach), such as the 'diamond press' and 'swan', will help to strengthen the trapezius and rhomboids. This, in turn, will help to strengthen the shoulder joint and shoulder girdle.

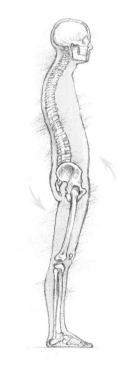

Above **Posterior pelvic tilt**

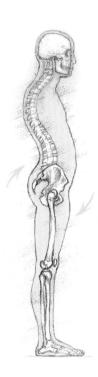

Above **Anterior pelvic tilt**

ROUND SHOULDERS SYNDROME

Round-shouldered posture deviates from the ideal in the following ways: usually, a protruding chin and cervical lordosis; the scapulae are placed forward on the ribcage, taking the shoulders in front of the body's plumbline; at the same time, the scapulae are pulled away from the ribcage into a 'winged position'.

This compromises movement as the muscle groups are unco-ordinated, with some muscles being shorter than others.

Round shoulder postural check list:
1. Head is level and ears are centered with the body's plumbline.
2. Open the shoulders without exaggerated contraction ('winging').
3. Palms face the sides of the body.
4. Elbows point backwards.

5. Open the pectorals and pull down the Lattisimus dorsi without visible winging of the scapulae.

PELVIC TILTING / LOWER BACK PLACEMENT

Pelvic tilting involves movement of the lower back and hip joints. The ideal pelvic placement – when the pelvis is in the neutral position (the hipbones and pubic bone are on the same plane) – is imperative to achieve the normal anterior curve of accurate lower back placement. See page 52 for how to locate the neutral pelvis.

a. Posterior pelvic tilt

The pelvis tilts backward, flattening the lumbar spine so there is no natural lordotic curve in the lower back. Stand in front of a mirror and tilt the pelvis into the neutral position to correct pelvic placement.

CROSS-TRAINING

Pilates exercises are excellent for cross-training purposes. The notion has always been that sporting activities develop strength, endurance, and flexibility. Now sportsmen and women need to develop muscular strength, endurance and flexibility in order to participate more effectively and safely – and they can do this using the Pilates programme of exercise.

Pilates does not necessarily have to replace a gym workout or other exercise or sporting activity. Using the knowledge gained through the Pilates system will enable you to make subtle, yet positive adaptations to your existing routine. The breathing and other Pilates principles and elements will improve your physical ability. A conscious approach to your physical

workout will change 'no brain movements' to conscious thinking movements. One important aspect to be addressed is the repetitive movement pattern that applies to your particular sport or workout.

A good example is golfing (right). The golf swing becomes a repetitive movement on one side of the body, often leading to back or shoulder problems. Runners frequently experience knee problems caused by incorrect knee and foot alignment and thus incorrect movement patterns. Many are unaware that by simply correcting their alignment through conscious understanding and effort, they could make their knee problems disappear.

Take into account the muscles that are utilized and overused in your programme

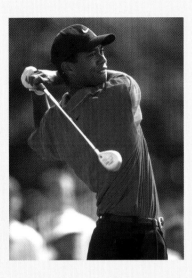

in order to select exercises that will stretch and strengthen the opposing muscles. Cross-training is an important aspect of total fitness, and is vital in strengthening all the muscles of the body to reduce muscle stress.

b. Anterior pelvic tilt or lordosis
This is an abnormal degree of arching of the lumbar spine. The pelvis tilts forward, decreasing the angle between the pelvis and the thigh. Stand in front of a mirror and tilt the pelvis into the neutral position to correct pelvic placement. Visualize tucking the tailbone between the legs.

MILITARY STANCE (EXTENDED RIBCAGE)
In the 'military type' posture, the ribcage is splayed, putting enormous tension on the back. Consciously softening the breastbone and placing the ribcage back into the body (the natural position of the ribcage when you exhale) will relax and improve this type of posture.

ABDOMINAL IMPORTANCE
The abdominal muscles play a critical role in keeping the spine erect and the body well lifted out of the hips. They spread horizontally, vertically and diagonally, wrapping the abdomen in sheets of tissue and creating a natural corset. On bending forward, they stabilize the spine from the front, co-contracting with the muscles of the back. As we bend, the abdominals provide the hydraulics for the precision of movement. The deepest abdominal muscle is the Transversus abdominis, which compresses the abdominals and stabilizes the back when you exhale. Pilates' 'belly to spine'

breathing engages this muscle to assist the spine, which is the body's strut. The Transversus abdominis lies close to the spine and is significantly targeted in all Pilates exercises as it provides a girdle of strength for the body.

With correctly developed abdominals, back-related problems can be improved as you develop greater strength and a more flattering waistline.

THE GOAL
The ultimate goal of Pilates is for you to understand the mechanics of your body and, as a result, to achieve conscious exercising within your own limits.

PILATES PRINCIPLES

ALTHOUGH today the classical Pilates exercises have been adapted to incorporate preparatory exercises suitable for people from all walks of life rather than only athletes and dancers, the principles have remained unchanged since Joseph Pilates incorporated them into his work.

The Pilates principles are:

1 Relaxation
2 Alignment
3 Breathing
4 The powerhouse or centre
5 Concentration
6 Co-ordination
7 Flowing movements
8 Stamina

These principles form the foundation of the Pilates technique and provide the key to deriving maximum benefit from the exercises. Take time to master them before embarking on the exercises. Remember that the quality of movement is always more important than the number of repetitions. The secret and power of Pilates lies in using the connections made through these principles.

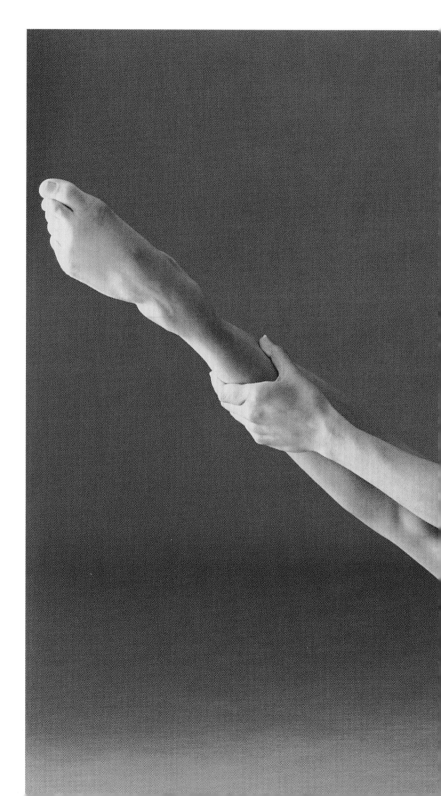

THE ESSENTIAL ELEMENTS

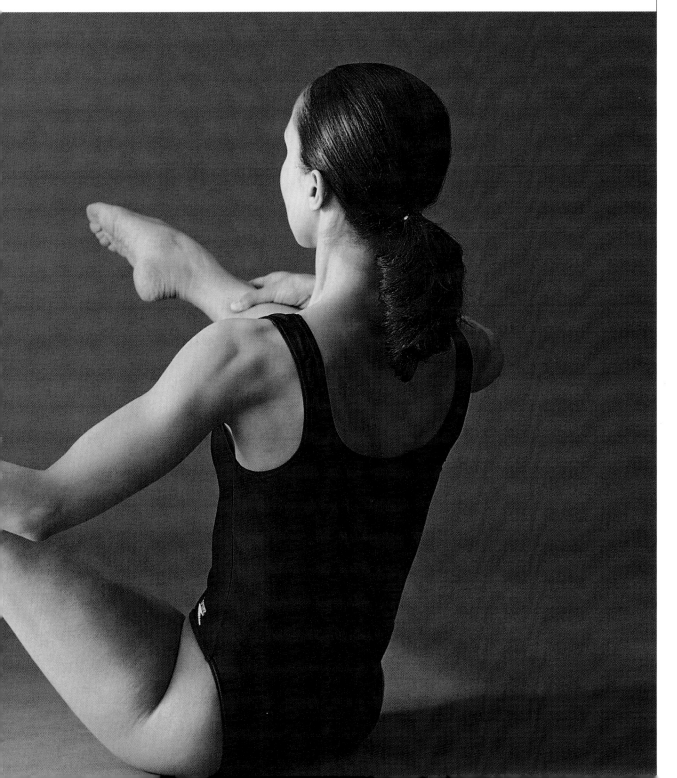

1 Relaxation

The balance between muscle tension and relaxation is often overlooked in exercise. The muscles need to be de-stressed before they are taken into exercise. Exercising tense muscles creates more tension, which can introduce inaccurate muscle functioning that ultimately defeats the object of the exercise.

In Pilates, pre-exercise relaxation is a prerequisite to any routine.

FOLLOW THE BREATH
Relaxation exercise

1. Lie on your back with knees flexed, soles of the feet on the mat, arms at your sides.
2. Close your eyes and relax all muscles in your body. Feel and relax the weight of the body into the floor.
3. Open the mouth, drop the jaw and move the tongue slightly to the back of the mouth.
4. Inhale and mentally focus to follow the breath as it enters the nose and travels into the lungs.
5. Exhale through the mouth. Mentally follow the breath as it leaves the body.
Breathe deeply on inhalation and exhalation. Concentrate only on the

breath; let all other thoughts slip away from your consciousness.

Visualization tip:

1. Paint the inhalation breath a blue colour. Follow the blue breath as it enters the nose right through to the lungs.
2. Paint the exhalation breath mauve. Follow the mauve breath as it leaves the lungs and exits through the mouth.

2 Alignment

The starting point of intelligent exercise is a correctly aligned body, with balanced muscles. Good alignment is when the muscles hold the joints in their natural position. The first step towards Pilates is addressing postural imbalances and working to correct and maintain balanced posture.

(a) Correct lower body alignment

- Draw an imaginary straight line vertically through the centre of the hip down to the centre of the kneecap, then down to the centre of the foot.
- The feet should not roll or turn inwards or outwards. When the lower body is misaligned it upsets upper body alignment as well, since

all parts of the body affect one another.

(b) Correct upper body alignment

Stabilize the scapula and shoulder girdle by ensuring that:

- The shoulders are not elevated but depressed.
- The shoulders do not pull forwards or backwards or 'wing'.
- Think and feel tall by growing through the tips of the ears, without shortening the back of the neck.
- Open the pectorals, lengthen the spine, pull down the Latissimus dorsi and pull the mid-back downwards to support the head correctly (without protruding or 'popping' the ribcage).

ALIGNMENT EXERCISE

1. Lie on your back with knees flexed, soles of the feet on the floor, legs hip-width apart, arms at your sides and elbows slightly bent.
2. Arch the back, gently roll the ribcage downwards and back into the body, and soften the breastbone. This takes the pelvis into the neutral position and maintains the natural lordotic curve of the lower back.
3. Engage the Latissimus dorsi. Feel the scapulae pulling down towards the hips.

Above **For the alignment exercise, people with increased curvature of the cervical spine (where the chin 'juts' forward) should place a folded towel or small cushion under the head to support the head and align the spine accurately.**

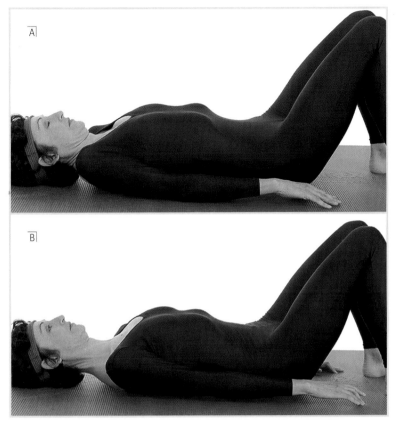

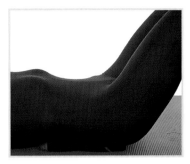

Above **People with increased lordosis should place a folded towel or small cushion under the lower back to support it and align the spine correctly.**

Exercise to engage the Latissimus dorsi

4. The head is in the neutral position, neither tilting forwards nor backwards.

Note:

- Always ensure the body is correctly aligned before starting an exercise.

EXERCISE TO ENGAGE THE LATISSIMUS DORSI

1. Lie on your back, knees flexed, soles of the feet on the mat, legs hip-width apart, arms at your sides and elbows slightly bent.

2. Shrug the shoulders up towards the ears (A). Walk the fingers down towards the toes (B) until the arms are fully extended. The shoulders are now released and depressed.

3. Feel the slight tension under the armpits and towards the back –

a sign that the Latissimus dorsi are engaging.

4. Hold onto the feeling of tension and bend the elbows slightly as in the starting position.

Breathing

'Millions have never learned to master the art of correct breathing.'
JOSEPH PILATES

In many exercise programmes the link between breathing and activity is unimportant. In Pilates, however, every movement is accompanied by active, conscious breathing.

The body needs oxygen to function optimally. Cell-building oxygen rushing through the arteries improves

circulation and releases pain and tension. Correct breathing during exercise relaxes the muscles. The Pilates breathing technique takes time to master and should be practised as often as possible. Keep your breathing continuous. Do not hold your breath as this wastes energy.

The Transversus abdominis muscle plays a major role in the correct breathing technique. On inhalation, the ribcage expands laterally and the diaphragm moves downwards. On exhalation, the lungs recoil and the diaphragm moves upwards to push air up and out. During forced expiration, the abdominals assist in this process. Visualize the belly button pulling further inwards towards the spine on every exhalation. In Pilates, inhalation usually accompanies spinal extension whereas exhalation usually accompanies spinal flexion.

In everyday life we do not utilize our breath effectively, but improved breathing patterns can release stress and increase stamina. Apply the breathing exercises in everyday life, as well as in the Pilates exercises.

BREATHING AND SUPPORT OF THE LOWER BACK

When the Transversus abdominis and obliques contract through exhalation, the lower back is supported and protected. The breathing technique, together with accurate neutral pelvic placement, is fundamental to the core stabilization process – and vital to anyone with back problems.

BREATHING AND TENSION

The neck and shoulders are particularly susceptible to tension, and can cause irritability and even ill health. Nothing is purely physical or mental, but psychophysical. Breathing is free when you are peaceful, but tense when you feel insecure. Correct breathing and conscious relaxation of the muscles of the back of the neck will help alleviate pain and tension.

BREATHING AND POSTURE

Posture has much to do with breathing habits. When the trunk is upright, the spine and muscles are correctly balanced. The diaphragm functions like a piston, creating a balanced action of tension and relaxation. Most people breathe shallowly, which inhibits proper functioning of the diaphragm and can cause health problems and ineffective functioning of abdominal muscles. Breathing should not only be about increasing oxygen inhalation, but about effective distribution.

Note:

- Inhale through the nose.
- Exhale through the mouth.
- Never hold the breath.
- Do not lift shoulders on inhalation.
- Always breathe laterally.

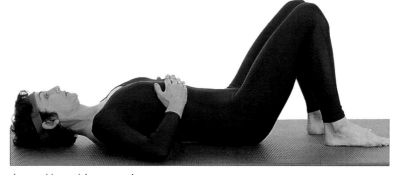

Lateral breathing exercise

- Always breathe rhythmically. The breathing pattern may have an adagio quality (long and slow) or a staccato quality (short and fast), depending on the exercise.
- Sustain the tension created in the abdominal cavity on exhalation ('belly to spine') for the next inhalation and throughout the exercise.

1. EXERCISE FOR LATERAL BREATHING

1. Lie on your back with knees flexed, hands on the ribcage.
2. On inhalation, feel the ribcage expanding **sideways** (instead of the chest rising up towards the shoulders).
3. On exhalation, feel the ribcage recovering and rolling back into the body.
4. Inhale for five seconds and exhale for five seconds. Build up eventually to inhale for eight seconds and exhale for eight seconds. This develops deep, slow breathing to fill the lungs fully on inhalation and fully deplete them on exhalation.

2. BREATHING THROUGH THE BACK

1. Sit on the mat, arms over your knees, bending the torso forward over the knees as shown below.
2. Consciously inhale then exhale, taking the breath only into the upper back. Repeat four or five times.
3. Now repeat the exercise but take the breath into the middle of the back. Repeat four or five times.
4. Repeat the exercise, this time breathing into the lower back. Repeat four or five times.

A partner or instructor may place his or her hands on your upper, middle and lower back to help you feel where you are taking the breath.

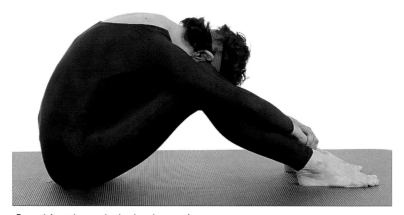

Breathing through the back exercise

3. STACCATO BREATHING

1. Lie on your back, hands on the abdomen, fingers towards the belly button.

2. Take six short, sharp sniffs through the nose, then exhale through the mouth with six short exhalations, as if blowing out six candles.

3. Retain the tension from the 'belly to spine' contraction in the abdominal cavity created by the Transversus abdominis and obliques when you exhale (i.e. after the first exhalation, do not release the abdominals at all on inhalation).

4. Repeat five to ten times.

Note:
- The Pilates breathing rule is: exhale and glue 'belly to spine' on effort. Apply this rule, too, to activities like climbing stairs or lifting heavy objects.

4 The powerhouse

Joseph Pilates believed the abdominals to be the 'powerhouse' of the body (also known as the girdle of strength or the centre). All movement is initiated from the centre, and equal strength is required between the abdominals and the back. People suffering from lower back pain usually lack abdominal strength. Pilates exercises work the deep Transversus abdominis and help to achieve a strengthened, flat abdomen.

In Pilates exercises all movement should be preceded by abdominal contraction. This means gluing the 'belly to spine' to stabilize pelvis and spine before starting a movement. Once the abdominals are engaged on exhalation, the pelvic floor or 'bathroom muscles' (used to stop urination) are also actively engaged.

PILLOW SQUEEZE EXERCISE

1. Lie on your back with knees flexed, arms at your sides, elbows slightly bent.

2. Place a small pillow between the knees.

3. Inhale through the nose for three counts.

4. Exhale through the mouth for three counts, squeezing the pillow between the knees. On the third count of the exhalation, activate the pelvic floor muscles.

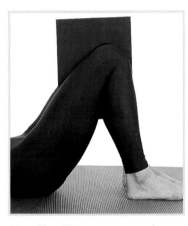

Above **The pillow squeeze exercise works the 'bathroom muscles' to help prevent incontinence.**

5 Concentration

'Always keep your mind wholly concentrated on the purpose of the exercises as you perform them.'
JOSEPH PILATES

It is only through concentration and the mind-body connection that you can detect and address hidden tensions and faulty movement patterns. Every movement should be a conscious act controlled by the mind. Taking the mind inside the spine requires focus and concentration.

The relaxation exercise at the beginning of this chapter will help set the right tone for the Pilates session. Thereafter, it takes determination and concentration to restrain random thoughts so that all your mental energy can be applied to the job at hand.

EXERCISE FOR CONCENTRATION AND FOCUS

1. Lie on your back, completely relaxed, with eyes closed.

2. Hear and listen to every sound you can possibly hear.

3. Focus only on sound.

4. Now concentrate on obliterating any other thoughts or images entering your mind.

5. Quietly retain your focus for about two minutes.

6 Co-ordination

'Start on the correct movements each time you exercise, lest you do them improperly and thus lose all the vital benefits of their value.'
JOSEPH PILATES

In Pilates, the entire body co-ordinates as a whole, instead of one part working in isolation. Breathing co-ordinates with the abdominals to stabilize the spine and pelvis before every movement. This develops the neuro-muscular ability to co-ordinate the mind and the body. Each exercise begins and ends with a conscious, co-ordinated breathing pattern. Each breath co-ordinates with a specific movement.

Achieving mind-body exercise requires concentration but is not difficult. Start with the easier exercises and enjoy the mental challenge.

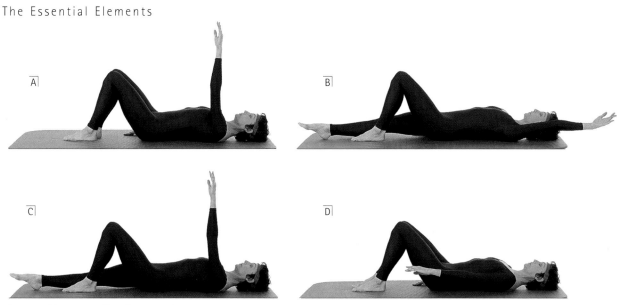

Arm and leg co-ordination exercise

ARM CO-ORDINATION EXERCISE

1. Lie on your back with knees bent, soles of the feet on the floor, legs hip-width apart, arms at your sides, elbows slightly bent and palms of the hands towards the floor.

2. Inhale through the nose and raise the left arm towards the ceiling.

3. Exhale to stabilize the abdominals, lower the left arm to the floor above your head, palm facing the ceiling. (Retain abdominal tension).

4. Inhale and raise the left arm upward towards the ceiling.

5. Exhale to stabilize the abdominals, and lower the left arm back down to the starting position.

Repeat the exercise with the right arm.

Repeat four times with each arm, alternating arms.

Points to remember about shoulder mobility:

• If shoulder mobility is limited, the arms should not be taken right back towards the floor. The lack of mobility will elevate the shoulders, which may cause tension.

• Take personal limitations into account and work within your personal range of movement.

• To avoid shoulder tension and elevation, feel the shoulder blades sliding down towards the hips as you raise and lower the arms.

LEG CO-ORDINATION EXERCISE

This exercise is the same as the arm co-ordination exercise but is now executed only with the legs. The starting position is the same.

1. Inhale.

2. Exhale – slide and extend the right leg just above the mat, opening the front of the hip on the full extension.

3. Inhale – hold the position.

4. Exhale – slide the right leg back to the starting position.

Repeat with the left leg.

Repeat the exercise four times with each leg, alternately.

Note:

• Aim to retain perfect pelvic stability throughout.

ARM AND LEG CO-ORDINATION EXERCISE

This exercise is a combination of the previous two exercises. The starting position is the same.

1. Inhale – raise the left arm upward towards the ceiling (A).

2. Exhale – slide the right leg down to extend along the mat. Simultaneously continue to extend the left arm backwards towards the floor (B). The leg and arm arrive at full extension at the same time as the end of the exhalation.

3. Inhale – raise the left arm back towards the ceiling (C).

3. Exhale – slide the right leg back towards the starting position and simultaneously continue moving the left arm back to the starting position (D). Both arm and leg complete their movements at the same time as the end of the exhalation.

4. Repeat four to six times, alternating sides.

Note:

• Try to secure perfect pelvic stability when the arm and leg start to move.

7 Movement

Movement is the greatest youth elixir. Freedom of movement empowers the body. With movement comes rhythm.

Pilates exercises incorporate naturally flowing, rhythmical movements. All movements should be executed with knowledge of the particular muscle or muscle group being targeted by the exercise. When movements are performed from a purely choreographic point of view, without deeper understanding, the exercise is ineffective.

At first, Pilates movements are slow and controlled, the principles consciously and carefully applied. More complex, more challenging exercises are introduced only when the principles are securely executed with flow and ease of movement. Only then should the pace of the session be increased.

Once the exercise starts there should be no beginning or end to the movements. Breathing is also considered as movement, where inhalation blends seamlessly into exhalation. The flowing movements of Pilates exercises require precision and fluidity, unlike the static, isolated movements of other exercise routines.

8 Stamina

Muscle imbalance and poor posture causes fatigue. When the stabilizing and mobilizing muscles work together as a team, backed by good breathing patterns, the body functions harmoniously. Uniformly developed muscles provide good posture, flexibility and grace so that energy is not wasted through inefficient movement. Instead, energy levels are increased and stamina is built.

CONTROL AND PRECISION

CONTROL

'Good posture can be successfully acquired only when the entire body is under perfect control.'
JOSEPH PILATES

Movements that are mechanical are not controlled. Control teaches you how to take charge. Pilates changes the way you think not only about exercise, but about everyday movement. Unconscious movements can lead to ineffective movement patterns, whereas controlled thinking becomes controlled movement. Without control, the efficiency of the exercise is reduced. One difficulty is to maintain control without tension. The flow and rhythm of Pilates movements help to relax the muscles without disengaging them. Control starts in the mind, which, in turn, activates the muscles.

PRECISION

'The benefits of Pilates depend solely on your performing the exercises exactly according to the instructions.'
JOSEPH PILATES

All Pilates movements are exact in their precision and exactly synchronized. If the movement becomes inaccurate (losing the connections of the applied principles), stop immediately, then restart the exercise and refocus with precision to achieve the emphasis and goal of the exercise.

ISOLATION

'Each muscle may co-operatively aid in the uniform development of all the other muscles.'
JOSEPH PILATES

Muscles are isolated only in theory. In practice, they work in groups. Learning and visualizing how the muscles work enhances your ability to understand both the goal of a particular exercise, and your own strengths and weaknesses. Identifying the various muscles working in combination with other muscles will improve the precision of your workout and your understanding of isolation.

ROUTINE

'Make up your mind that you will perform your Pilates movements ten minutes each day without fail.'
JOSEPH PILATES

Routine is one part physical exertion and three parts self discipline. Infrequent exercise with minimal demands placed on the body will not deliver results. Put aside time for your session. It takes discipline to change your shape, your habits and your thinking. Routinely working all the muscles, changing and interchanging the movements, builds stamina. Only through practice will you reap the physical and mental benefits.

Preparing for your Pilates session

WORKING *out at a Pilates studio is the ideal. If you exercise at a studio and do additional exercises at home you will achieve your goals much sooner. If you cannot attend classes at a studio, however, create your own Pilates space at home.*

Suggested warm-up routine

1. Breathing and visualization
2. Elevation and depression
3. Protraction and retraction
4. Crossing elbows
5. Elbow circles
6. The Cossack
7. The dumb waiter

Suggested stretching routine

1. Easy hip stretch
2. Easy groin stretch
3. Easy shoulder stretch
4. Easy hip flexor stretch
5. Easy hamstring stretch

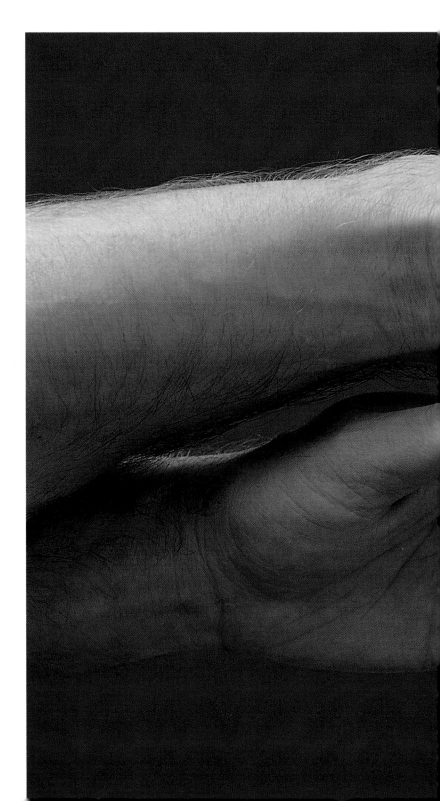

WARMING UP

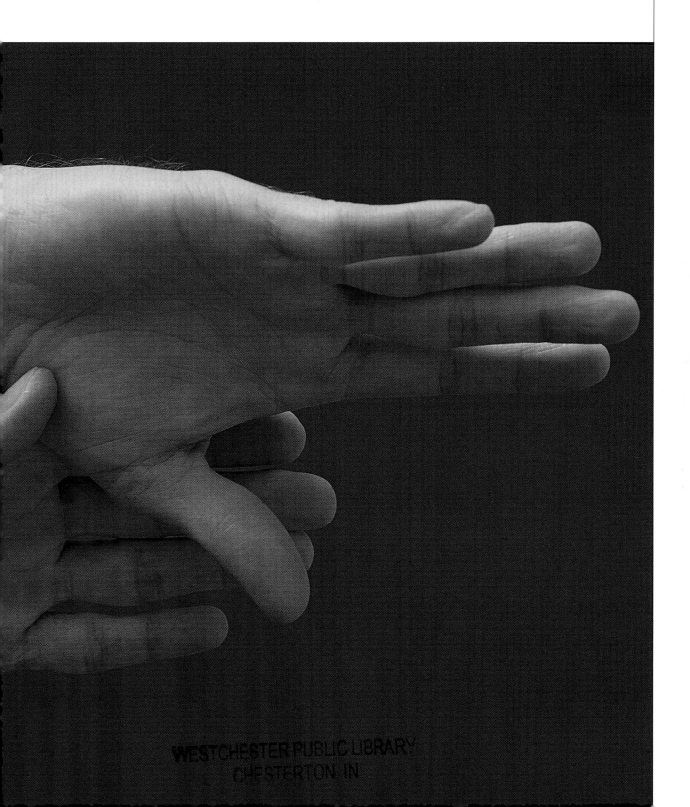

SETTING THE TONE

At home, it is important to work in a space free of noise and disturbance, although you do not have to exercise in total silence. Soft, soothing music in the background could add to the mood of your session.

To complete a balanced class takes about an hour. Pilates exercise is not aerobic at first,

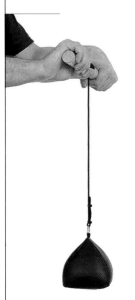

so it is advisable to incorporate brisk walking, running or cycling on an exercise bicycle into your routine to raise your heart rate.

For an effective, safe workout, the room in which you exercise should be at a comfortable temperature, and you should wear clothing that does not restrict your movements.

It is essential to invest in a good exercise mat. Hand or ankle weights

are optional extras. If you choose to use weights, ensure they are not too heavy for your ability. Start with light weights to avoid strain and tension, increasing them only once you master the exercise using the Pilates principles. If weights are too heavy, the mobilizing muscles take over and the stabilizing muscles do not work effectively – defeating the aim of Pilates.

If you tend to 'jut' your neck forward you will need a folded towel or small pillow as a neck support for most supine exercises. Those with an increased lordosis need a small pillow or folded towel for lower back support in the supine position.

PHYSICAL PROBLEMS

If you are fortunate enough to have a Pilates tutor, enlighten him or her about any physical problems you have, or have had previously. This enables the teacher to identify the weak areas of your body and choose suitable exercises for your condition

and ability. It is to your advantage to attend classes with an experienced teacher if you have had back surgery, prolapsed disc problems, osteoporosis, or if you are pregnant. Exercises incorporating full forward flexion and lateral flexion and rotation of the spine should be avoided if you have osteoporosis, prolapsed disc problems or a spinal fusion. Learn which exercises are appropriate for you before embarking on an exercise programme by yourself at home.

CHOICE OF EXERCISES

Always start with a warm-up routine. Warm-ups are not non-exercises and should not be treated as such. They are designed to relax and loosen the tight areas of your body, and are part of the mind-body preparation for the session ahead. The routine is designed to work the body in a supine (on your back), prone (on your stomach) and side position, incorporating spinal flexion, spinal extension and lateral spinal flexion to work the entire range of the spine.

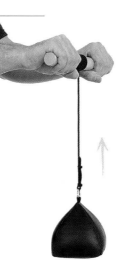
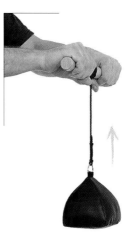
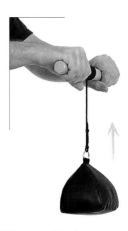

Left **Lifting a weight bag by 'rolling' the wrists strengthens arms and wrists.**

Always listen to your body. Pain is the body's way of telling you that you are in a 'no go' area so avoid any exercise that takes you into a stressed area of your body. Rather analyze why that particular area is stressed and identify what you can do about it.

Do not confuse discomfort with pain. If you are doing Pilates for the first time, your muscles will be experiencing new movement patterns and may rebel against the unfamiliar action. If an exercise is very uncomfortable, ask your instructor to reduce the intensity or adjust the exercise to a more preparatory level. Once the required strength is achieved, it will be easy to move to the next level.

Pilates exercises are not easy. The simplest exercise requires concentration, precision, control, co-ordination and isolation. This means, however, that the routine is never boring.

Should you lose the 'powerhouse' or neutral spine connection (see page 52), stop, think, and restart the exercise. Remember that the exercises lose their value when the connections are lost or if the routine is rushed. Work at your own pace and within your range of movement and ability. When you have strengthened sufficiently in the 'step-by-step' routine, the more advanced exercises present a further challenge. Follow the suggested repetitions for each exercise, remembering that Pilates is not about quantity of repetitions, but precision.

Right **Floor equipment like the barrel can be used to 'release' and open the back.**

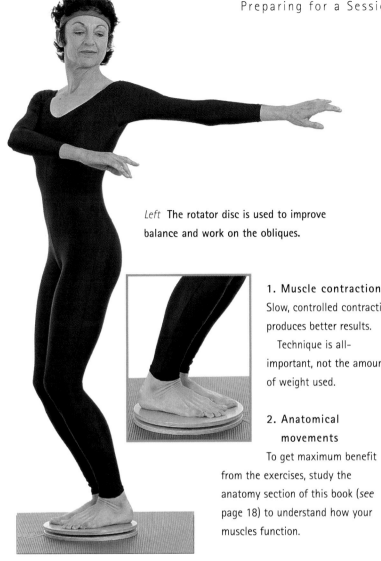

Left **The rotator disc is used to improve balance and work on the obliques.**

Your progress will depend on your commitment to mastering the Pilates technique. You can do anything to which you set your mind.

Always bear the following points in mind as you exercise:

1. Muscle contraction
Slow, controlled contraction produces better results.

Technique is all-important, not the amount of weight used.

2. Anatomical movements
To get maximum benefit from the exercises, study the anatomy section of this book (see page 18) to understand how your muscles function.

3. Good posture is vital
The pelvic position affects the lumbar spine, which, in turn, can affect the thoracic and cervical spine.

Work from the neutral position of the pelvis and retain correct shoulder placement.

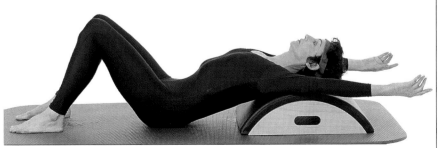

SUGGESTED WARM-UP ROUTINE

WARM-UP exercises are a pre-requisite to the routine. They limber and warm the body to improve the blood flow from the heart to the muscles and prepare them for the more demanding work ahead.

Simple warm-up exercises are a perfect mental preparation for the precise, accurately co-ordinated movements the Pilates routine demands. Use the warm-up time to focus on the self and to shut out the events of the day.

All the suggested exercises may be executed:
- sitting on an exercise ball
- sitting on a chair
- sitting cross legged on the floor, or
- standing upright with good posture.

1 Breathing and visualization

Breathing exercises help to regroup, harness and restore the energy. Use the relaxation exercise 'Follow the Breath' (see 'Pilates principles' on page 34) as the first warm-up exercise of your routine.

2 Elevation and depression

8–10 repetitions
Releases neck and upper body tension.
Starting position
Sit tall with your arms relaxed at your sides.

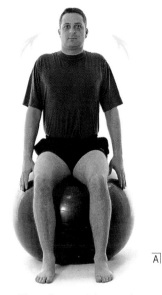
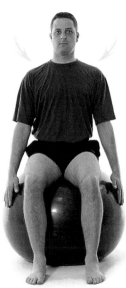

Elevation and depression

Exercise
Inhale – shrug your shoulders towards your ears (A).
Exhale – pull your shoulders down towards your hips (B).
Muscular emphasis
Upper trapezius (shoulder elevation); Latissimus dorsi (shoulder depression); Transversus abdominis and obliques (exhalation)

3 Protraction and retraction

8–10 repetitions
(one protraction plus one retraction = one repetition)
Starting position
Lift arms to shoulder height in front of you and retain this arm position throughout. Do not lift your shoulders.
Exercise
Inhale.
Exhale – reach the arms forward to

pull shoulders forward and away from the spine (A).
Inhale – release shoulders back to the starting position.
Exhale – retract shoulders, i.e. pull them back towards the spine (B).
Inhale – release shoulders to the starting position.
Muscular emphasis
Transversus abdominis, obliques (exhalation); rhomboids; Serratus anterior (protraction); mid trapezius (retraction)

4 Crossing elbows

6 repetitions (3 to each side)
Starting position
Place the right arm, bent at the elbow, in front of your face with your palm facing you. Lock the left elbow behind the right elbow (A).
Exercise
Inhale.

Exhale – raise both arms upward with elbows locked. Hold the position for five to eight seconds (B).
Release arms to repeat exercise on other side.

Muscular emphasis
Trapezius (lifting arms up); Transversus abdominis, obliques (exhalation)

Elbow circles
10 repetitions each way
Starting position
Place fingertips on your shoulders but do not lift your shoulders (A). Circle elbows 10 times in one direction (B, C, D), then reverse to circle 10 times in the other direction. (Make elbow rotations small to avoid lifting shoulders.)
Exercise
Inhale on the first half of rotation and exhale on the second half.
Muscular emphasis
Transversus abdominis and obliques (exhalation); deltoids; pectorals; rotator cuff muscles; shoulder and scapulae stabilizers; biceps

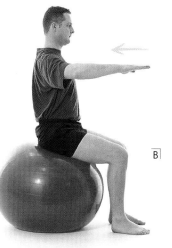 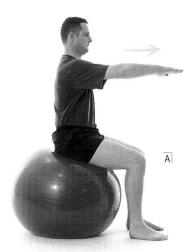

Protraction and retraction

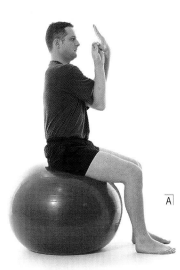 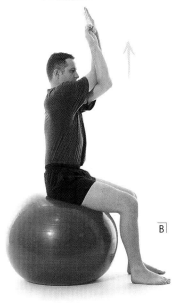

Crossing elbows

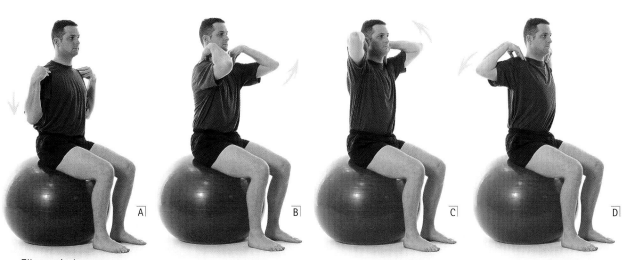

Elbow circles

6 The Cossack

6–10 repetitions, alternate sides

Starting position

Place arms at breastbone level, right hand on top of the left elbow, right elbow on top of the left hand (A).

Exercise

Inhale.

Exhale – rotate upper body to the right without moving hips or allowing ribs to pop forward (B).

Inhale – retain the position.

Exhale – return to starting position, extending and growing taller from the base of spine (A).

Repeat on the other side.

Visualization

Arms are held as in a Cossack dance.

Muscular emphasis

Transversus abdominis and obliques (exhalation); internal and external obliques; multifidi; Erector spinae

7 The dumb waiter

6–8 repetitions

Starting position

Place elbows into the sides of the waist with palms facing upwards and fingers together (A).

Exercise

Inhale.

Exhale – open the lower part of the arms sideways, retaining elbow into waist placement (B). Now apply resistance by pulling thumbs backwards and simultaneously pulling elbows forwards. Hold the position.

Inhale – return arms to the starting position (A).

Visualization

Start as if balancing a tea tray on the palms of the hands. Once the arms are opened sideways, visualize

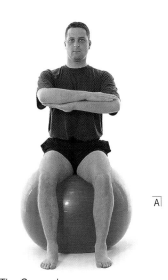
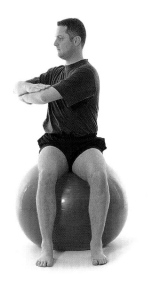

The Cossack

invisible gnomes pulling the thumbs backwards while others pull the elbows forwards to create resistance.

Muscular emphasis

Transversus abdominis (exhalation); deltoids; biceps; rotator cuff muscles

Note:

- It is the resistance that makes the exercise effective.
- Take care to retain the elbow into waist placement throughout the exercise.

ADDITIONAL WARM-UP EXERCISES:

1. Marching on the spot: 60–100 marches.

2. Hops on the spot: 20–60 hops.

3. Swinging the arms forwards and backwards, and sideways: 20 repetitions.

4. Cycling: 20 repetitions each way. Lie on your back with spine imprinted and both legs in the air. Cycle the legs in the air, then reverse rotation as if peddling backwards.

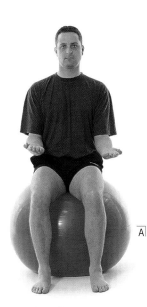
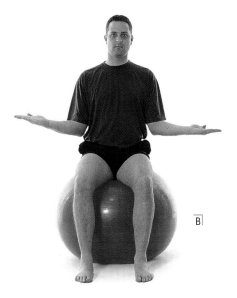

The dumb waiter

SUGGESTED STRETCHING ROUTINE

THE stretches in this section may be included as part of the warm-up routine to awaken the body and make you feel good.

Note:

- Strive to hold the stretches for about two minutes and incorporate the Pilates principles.
- Counter-stretching is important so that muscles do not become over-strained.
- Avoid selecting exercises that concentrate only on a specific area of the body. Hip extensor stretches should be counter-balanced with hip flexor stretches and vice versa; spinal flexion exercises should follow spinal extension exercises and vice versa.
- Use the breath and on the stretch exhale into the particular area being stretched.

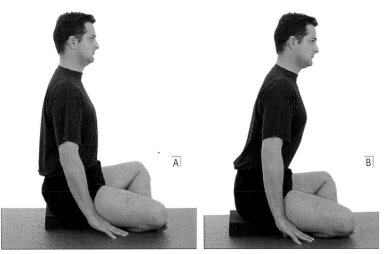

Easy hip stretch

1 Easy hip stretch
2–6 repetitions

1. Sit on a cushion with legs crossed in front, feet slightly in front of the knees so the lower half of the leg is at 90 degrees in front of you (A).

2. Lengthen the spine, lifting the breastbone upwards, then lean forward (B).
3. Relax into hip area of body.
4. Hold for 30 seconds to two minutes, feeling the stretch in the buttock and outer thigh.

2 Easy groin stretch
2–6 repetitions

1. Sit on a cushion with your back against the wall, knees dropped towards the floor, soles of the feet together.
2. Lengthen and straighten your back against the wall.
3. Allow your knees to drop even more to the floor.
4. Lift chest upwards without 'popping' the ribcage.
5. Hold for 30 seconds to two minutes, feeling the stretch in the adductors (groin).

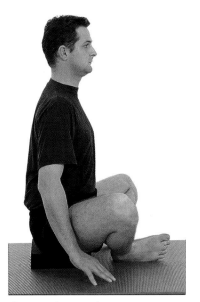

Easy groin stretch

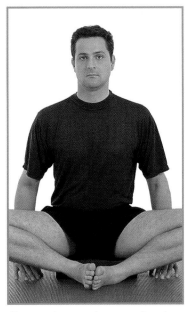

Easy groin stretch – anterior view

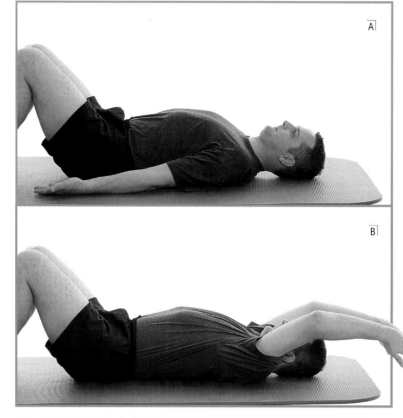

Easy shoulder stretch A

3 Easy shoulder stretch A
6 repetitions

1. Lie on your back on the mat with knees bent and arms at your sides, palms facing towards the ceiling (A).
2. Lift arms backwards overhead so the palms face down towards the floor and are externally rotated (B). Do not lift the shoulders or allow the ribcage to 'pop'.
3. Hold for 30 seconds to two minutes.
4. Return to the starting position.
Note:
- Ensure accurate scapular placement (shoulder blades sliding down towards the hips as the arms travel overhead).
  - Avoid arching the lower back or letting the ribcage 'pop'.
- Take the arms back only as far as you can while retaining accurate shoulder placement.

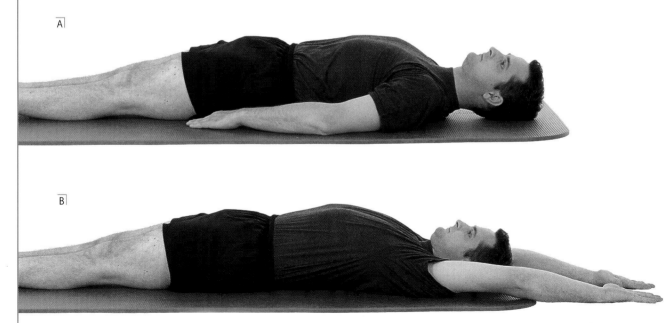

Easy shoulder stretch B

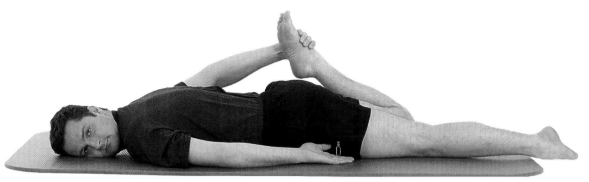

Easy hip flexor stretch

Easy shoulder stretch B

4 repetitions

1. Lie on your back on the mat, with your legs straight, arms at your sides, palms facing the floor (A).

2. Take the arms overhead towards the floor to finish with palms facing upwards (B). Extend and tighten front thighs to keep legs firmly down. Feel the stretch in the back of the shoulders.

3. Hold for 30 seconds to two minutes.

Note:

* Apply accurate scapular placement (shoulder blades sliding down towards the hips as the arms travel overhead).

* Apply accurate ribcage placement (do not let the ribcage 'pop').

Easy hip flexor stretch

2–6 repetitions, alternating sides

1. Lie on your stomach on the mat.

2. Pull one foot up towards the buttocks with your hand.

3. Ensure knee is in line with the hip.

4. Pull the heel slightly to the outside of the buttock.

5. Pull the front ribs slightly in to avoid arching your back.

6. Hold for 30 seconds to two minutes, feeling the stretch in the front of the thigh.

7. Repeat with the other foot.

Note:

* Using a small cushion under the pelvis releases lower back tension.

Easy hamstring stretch

2–4 repetitions, alternating sides

1. Lie on your back with legs up against a wall, arms at your sides.

2. Allow the buttocks to drop downwards to get the pubic bone in line with the belly button.

3. Stretch knees and front of the thighs and pull toes downwards. If the hamstrings are very tight, move the buttocks away from the wall slightly as shown.

4. Hold for 30 seconds to two minutes, feeling the stretch at the back of the thighs.

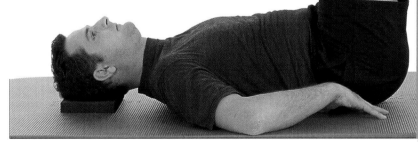

Easy hamstring stretch

Step-by-step exercises

The more advanced routine

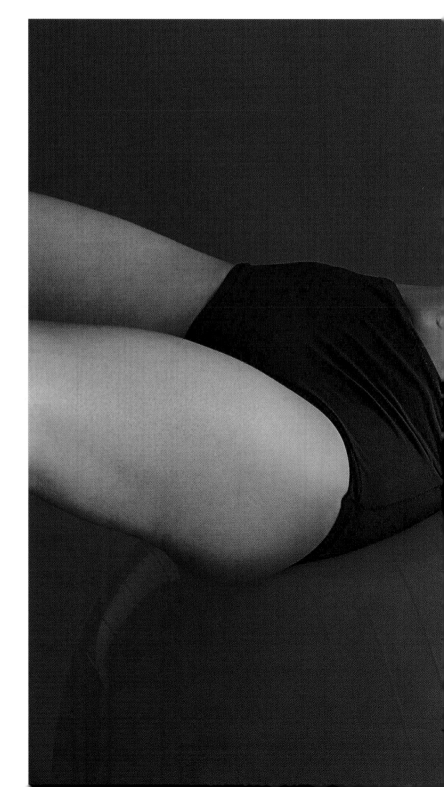

A BALANCED SESSION

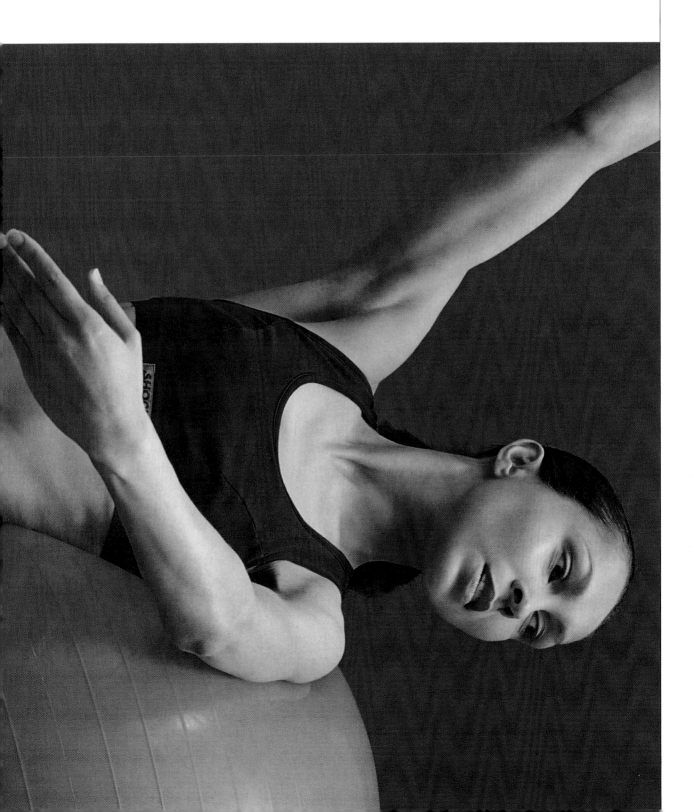

STEP-BY-STEP EXERCISES

THE exercises should be performed in the correct order to provide a balanced session. Always assume the correct position before starting an exercise. Begin with the easier, preparatory exercises before attempting more difficult exercises. Remember that it takes time to develop strength and to understand each exercise. Read the instructions carefully and employ the detail when executing each exercise.

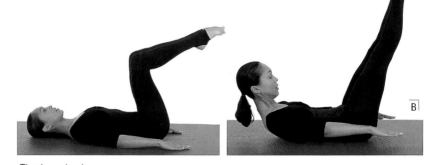

The hundred

1 The hundred

10 repetitions (100 counts)
Increases circulation.
Breathing and endurance exercise.
Co-ordinates breathing with movement.

Starting position
Lie on your back on the mat with knees bent, legs in the air, spine imprinted, inner thighs connected, arms at your sides (A).

Exercise
Inhale – to 'nod'.
Exhale – flex the upper body off the

mat, reach arms slightly off the mat and extend legs fully (B).
Inhale for five counts and exhale for five counts, pulsing the arms up and down. Take the movement from the shoulder joint, emphasizing the downward pulse.
Keep the Latissimus dorsi engaged to achieve the desired control.

Ending
Inhale – hold the position.
Exhale – lower the head, then lower the legs one at a time.

Visualization
Wrists hammering nails into the floor boards.

Muscular emphasis
Abdominals; hip flexors; Latissimus dorsi

Note:
- Retain abdominal tension.
- Avoid neck strain.
- Retain imprinted spine.

PREPARATORY EXERCISE A:
10 repetitions (100 counts)
Starting position
As in the main exercise, but keep your feet on the ground, legs hip-width apart, knees bent, soles of feet on the mat.
Exercise
Remain in the starting position, working on breathing and arm movements as in the main exercise.

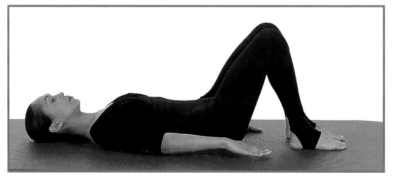

The hundred – preparatory exercise A

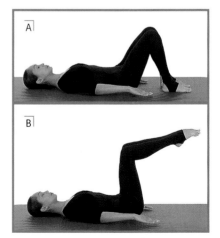

The hundred – preparatory exercise B

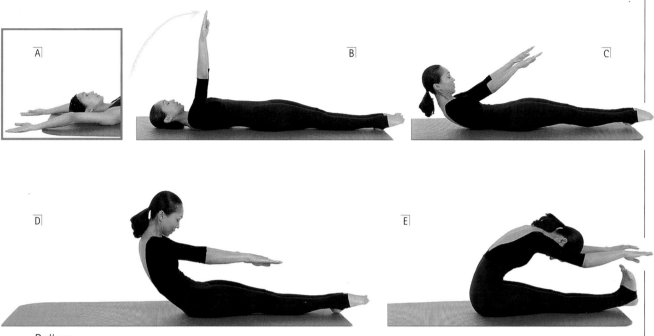

Roll up

PREPARATORY EXERCISE B:
10 repetitions (100 counts)

Starting position
As in preparatory exercise A (A).

Exercise
Raise legs together in the air, knees above hips, but not fully extended (B). Breathing and ending are as for the main exercise.

2 Roll up
5–10 repetitions
Spine extensor stretch accenting use of the abdominals.

Starting position
Lie on your back on the mat, arms above your head (A), legs extended, inner thighs connected, pelvis neutral.

Exercise
Inhale – reach arms forward towards the ceiling (B) and 'nod' (C). Exhale – roll your spine up off mat (D), one vertebra at a time, until your arms are parallel with the floor. Now dorsi-flex the feet (E). Inhale – roll back, one vertebra at a time, until you reach the hinge position at the hips (D). Exhale – complete the roll down, taking arms above the head back to the starting position (A).

Visualization
Roll and unroll the body like a Swiss roll cake.

Muscular emphasis
Abdominals; hip flexors; hamstrings; shoulder girdle stabilizers

Note:
- Individuals who have a vulnerable lower back and weak abdominals should do the preparatory exercise instead.
- Avoid shoulder elevation and tension.
- Take care not to jam or jut your chin forward.

PREPARATORY EXERCISE:
4 repetitions
Flex the upper body off the mat and pulse five times.

Starting position
As in full exercise but with arms at your sides.

Exercise
Inhale – to 'nod'.
Exhale – flex upper body off the mat.
Inhale.

Exhale – pulse the body forward five times as you exhale (use one short exhalation for each forward pulse).

Ending
Inhale.
Exhale – roll back down towards the floor to the starting position.

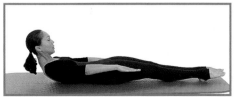

Roll up – preparatory exercise

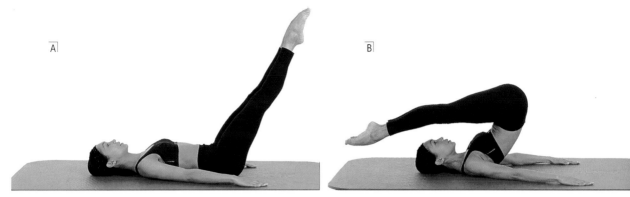

Roll over

3

Roll over

4 repetitions each way
(To be avoided by those with neck or lower back problems)
Increases flexibility and strength in the back, and strengthens abdominals and shoulders.

Starting position

Lie on your back on the mat, arms at your sides, legs extended together in the air. Lower your legs as far as possible, retaining imprinted spine, and contract the abdominals (A).

Exercise

Inhale – take legs backward to hinge at the hip and stretch to lengthen the hamstrings (back of the legs).

Exhale – roll your spine off the mat and send your legs overhead towards the floor (B).

Inhale – open the legs hip-distance apart and dorsi-flex the feet (C).

Exhale – roll back down through the spine and onto the mat (D). Bring the legs together in the air to restart (A). Reverse the exercise to roll backwards with legs hip-distance apart. After four repetitions, roll back down towards the mat with inner thighs squeezed together and feet dorsi-flexed.

Visualization

Simulate the controlled action of each vertebra to the movement of a clock's second hand – one 'tick' at a time, and one vertebra at a time.

Muscular emphasis

Abdominals; hamstrings; hip flexors; shoulder girdle stabilizers

Note:

- Sustain abdominal contraction when exhaling.
- Control the articulation of the vertebra as the spine peels off and back on to the mat.

PREPARATORY EXERCISE:

Hold onto the back of the legs and send them backwards in a rocking motion, lifting the tailbone off the floor. Flex legs at the knees at first, then work towards extending them.

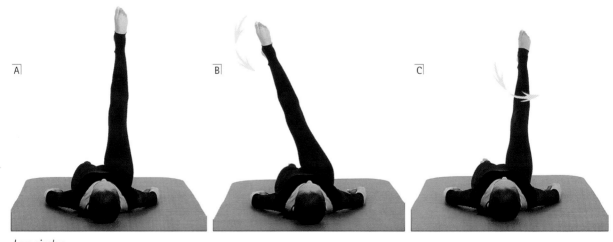

Leg circles

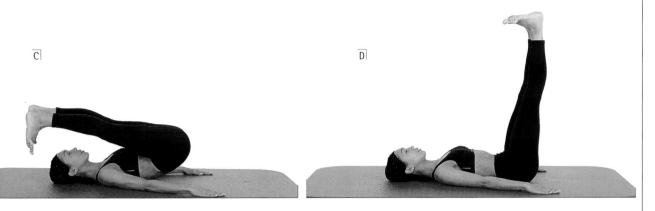

C | D |

4 Leg circles

5 circles each way
Lubricates ball and socket joint in the
hip, and loosens the hip.
Stretches the hamstrings.

Starting position
Lie on your back with one leg
extended along the mat and the
other extended in the air at a
90-degree angle, arms at your sides
and neutral pelvis (A).

Exercise
Inhale – trace half a circle in the air
with the foot (B, C).
Exhale – trace the other half of the
circle with the foot (D, A).
Pause after each circle to stabilize.

Visualization
An oval football.

Muscular emphasis
Abdominals, especially obliques;
hamstrings; quadriceps; adductors

Note:
- Avoid upper body tension or
  sideways movement of the pelvis.
- Dorsi-flex or point the foot in the air.

PREPARATORY EXERCISES:
(For individuals with tight hamstrings
and hip flexors)

EXERCISE A
As for main exercise, but bend both
knees.

EXERCISE B
As in main exercise, but extend the leg
on the mat and bend the leg in the air.

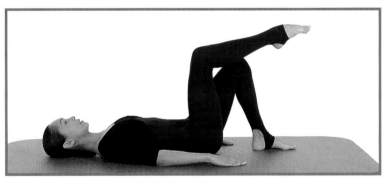

Leg circles – preparatory exercise A

D |

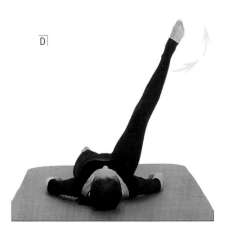

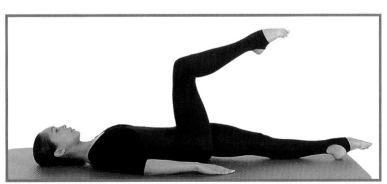

Leg circles – preparatory exercise B

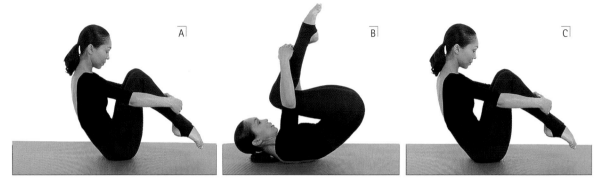

Rolling like a ball

5 Rolling like a ball

10 repetitions
Increases mobility and balance.
Improves abdominal control.

Starting position
Sit on the mat just off the sitting bones, legs together, knees flexed towards your chest. Raise feet off the mat, hands on shins, abdominals and spine in a C-curve. Take eye line towards the knees (A).

Exercise
Inhale – retain C-curve and rock backwards (B).
Exhale – rock back up to the starting position to balance just back off the sitting bones, retaining the C-curve (C).

Visualization
The base of a rocking horse.

Muscular emphasis
Hamstrings; gluteus muscles; hip flexors; hip adductors; shoulder girdle stabilizers; abdominals

Note:
- Avoid losing the C-curve.
- Relax the shoulders.

PREPARATORY EXERCISE A:
10 repetitions
Starting position as in the main exercise. Balance on the sitting bones (A). On inhalation, move the torso away from the thigh (B), then move back towards the thigh on exhalation. Retain the C-curve throughout.

PREPARATORY EXERCISE B:
10 repetitions
Start as in the main exercise. First, practise the rocking motion without stopping to balance. Then add the breathing pattern as in the main exercise.

6 Single leg stretch

10–20 sets
Improves co-ordination.
Builds strength.

Starting position
Lie on your back on the mat with legs in the air, knees bent, inner thighs connected, hands holding sides of the knees. Spine should be imprinted.
Inhale – to 'nod'.
Exhale – lift upper torso off the mat (A).

Exercise
Inhale.
Exhale – extend one leg, then interchange to extend the other leg while bending the first. Take the outside hand towards the ankle of the shortened leg and inside hand to the inside of the bent knee (B).
Inhale – retain spinal flexion and switch legs twice (one set).
Exhale – retain spinal flexion and

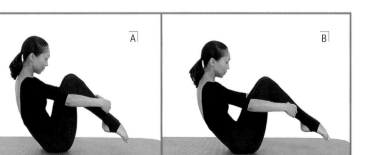

Rolling like a ball – preparatory exercise A

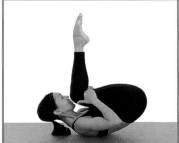

Preparatory exercise B

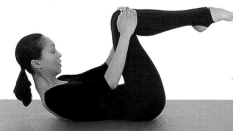

Single leg stretch

switch legs twice (one set). When right leg is lengthened, the left arm is lengthened, and vice versa.

Ending

Inhale. Exhale and lower the head and one leg, then lower the other leg.

Visualization

A piston action.

Muscular emphasis

Abdominals; hamstrings; hip flexors; quadriceps (thighs); shoulder girdle stabilizers

Note:

• Avoid neck tension or losing the spinal imprint.

• Retain abdominal contraction throughout.

PREPARATORY EXERCISE:

10 repetitions

Start as in the main exercise. Support the back of the head with the hands and do one exhalation per leg extension. Inhale when legs are bent together; exhale as one leg extends.

7 Side to side obliques

10–20 sets

(For individuals with lower back problems or whose abdominal strength requires more development, keep feet on the mat and knees bent.)

Builds abdominal strength.

Starting position

Lie on your back on the mat with legs in the air, inner thighs connected, knees bent, imprinted spine, hands supporting the back of the head (A).

Exercise

Inhale – to 'nod'.

Exhale – stretch one leg and obliquely twist the body towards the bent leg, then switch legs – one set (B, C).

Inhale – switch legs twice and obliquely twist the body towards the bent leg (B, C).

Exhale – switch legs twice and obliquely twist the body towards the bent leg (B, C).

Ending

Inhale – bring knees together in the air.

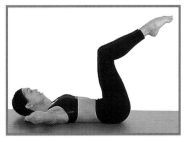

Single leg stretch – preparatory exercise

Exhale – lower the head, then lower the legs one at a time.

Visualization

The arms are like the wings of an aeroplane banking to the side.

Muscular emphasis

Abdominals, especially obliques; hamstrings; quadriceps; hip flexors; shoulder girdle stabilizers

Note:

• Aim for a slight side bend, with slight oblique forward twist. Take care not to side bend only.

• Avoid neck tension.

• Stay imprinted and retain abdominal contraction.

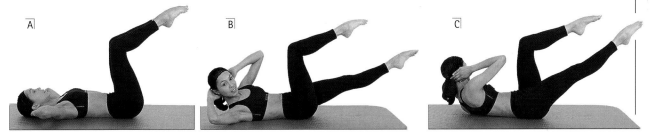

Side to side obliques

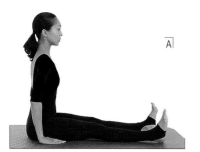
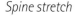
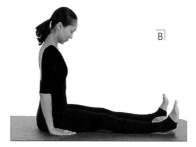
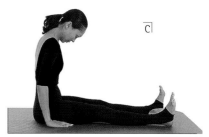

Spine stretch

8 Spine stretch

5 repetitions

Stretches and lengthens the spine to create space between the vertebrae.

Starting position

Sit tall with neutral spine, legs extended and spaced apart just wider than the shoulders. Feet are dorsi-flexed, arms rest on the floor slightly in front of the body (A).

Exercise

Inhale – lengthen upwards from the base of the spine.

Exhale – peel spine downwards, articulating one vertebra at a time (B, C, D).

Inhale – retain full forward flexion and breathe into the back (D).

Exhale – return to the starting position, articulating one vertebra at a time (D, C, B, A).

Visualization

Sinking down – spinal flexion.

Climbing up a ladder one step or 'one vertebra' at a time – spinal extension.

Muscular emphasis

Abdominals; Erector spinae; multifidi

Note:

- Do not jam your chin onto your chest.
- Avoid backward or forward pelvic tilt.

PREPARATORY EXERCISE:

5 repetitions

(Individuals with tight lower backs, hamstrings and hip flexors should sit on a firm pillow.)

The exercise is the same as the main exercise but executed with the feet together, the legs bent and laterally rotated.

9 The saw

5 repetitions each side, alternating

Improves mobility.

Stretches the upper back.

Starting position

Sit tall, spine in neutral, legs extended just wider than shoulders, feet dorsi-flexed, arms lifted to either side of the body just below shoulder height, palms facing forward (A). Avoid lifting hands higher than the shoulders.

Exercise

Inhale – rotate spine to the right, reach arms diagonally, keeping hips to the front (B).

Exhale – reach the left hand towards the right baby toe and turn palm of the back hand towards the spine (C).

Inhale – roll up through the spine, retain spinal rotation, turn palm of the hand away from the spine (D).

Exhale – return to starting position (E).

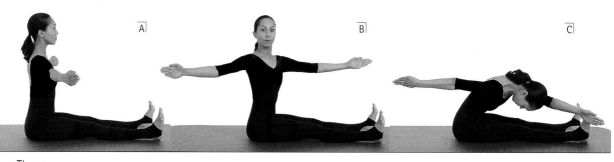

The saw

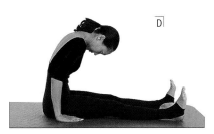

Repeat on the other side.

Visualization

The arm reaches forward to saw off the little toe.

Muscular emphasis

Obliques; multifidi; Erector spinae; Quadratus lumborum; shoulder girdle stabilizers

Note:

- Do not allow the opposite hip to lift during the forward stretch.
- Retain abdominal contraction throughout.

PREPARATORY EXERCISE:

5 repetitions
(For individuals with tight lower backs, hamstrings and hip flexors)
As in the main exercise but sit on a pillow and allow the knees to bend.

10 Diamond press

6–8 repetitions
Strengthens the upper back.

Starting position

Lie on your stomach on the mat with legs extended, inner thighs connected, elbows bent, forehead resting on your hands between the thumbs and first fingers (pointers). Place the thumbs and first pointers together to make a diamond shape (A).

Exercise

Inhale – lengthen the spine.
Exhale – glue hands to the forehead and float hands and elbows off the mat – not too high (B). Retain the lengthened line of the spine and do not look upward.
Inhale – sustain the position in the air (B).
Exhale – lower hands and elbows to the starting position (A).

Visualization

Stay lengthened and long as a dart.

Muscular emphasis

Abdominals; trapezius; Quadratus lumborum; neck extensors; adductors (inner thighs)

Note:

- Those with kyphosis-type posture (rounded back) may place a pillow

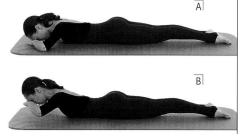

Diamond press

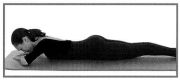

Preparatory exercise B

under the chest for support to try to achieve a neutral spine.
- Open the front of the chest and the back.
- Retain accurate head placement and avoid neck tension.
- Take care not to form 'wings' (press shoulder blades together).
- Pull bottom rib inwards.

PREPARATORY EXERCISE A:

5 repetitions

Starting position

As in the main exercise.

Exercise

Practise 'belly to spine' breathing (*see page 37*).

PREPARATORY EXERCISE B:

6 repetitions

Starting position

As in the main exercise.

Exercise

On exhalation, float only the head off the hands.

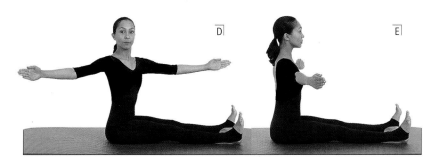

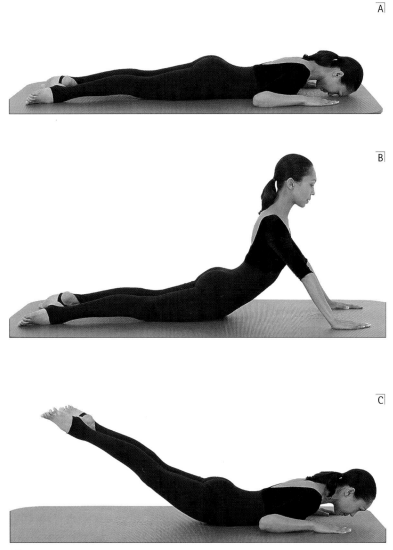

The swan

11

The swan

5 repetitions
Strengthens the back, neck and shoulders.

Starting position

Lie on your stomach on the mat, with legs lengthened, turned outwards and slightly apart, arms bent at the elbows, hands between the shoulders and ears, palms and forehead on the mat (A).

Exercise

Inhale – push the body upward with the arms to extend the spine (B).
Exhale – lower the body down towards the mat, rocking onto the upper torso and extending the legs behind you as they come up off the mat (C).

Ending

Inhale – push the body upward with the arms to extend the spine.
Exhale – lower body down to floor (A).

Visualization

The base of a rocking horse.

Muscular emphasis

Shoulder girdle stabilizers; Latissimus dorsi; Quadratus lumborum; gluteus muscles; abdominals; hamstrings

Note:

- Avoid tension in the upper trapezius.
- Try not to over-use the back and neck extensor muscles.
- Avoid this exercise if you have lower back problems.

PREPARATORY EXERCISE:

5 repetitions

Starting position

As in the main exercise.

Exercise

The legs do not leave the mat. Use four breaths as follows:
Inhale.
Exhale – push the body up to extend the spine.
Inhale – maintain extension.
Exhale – return to the starting position.

Advanced swan – rock and catch

(Instructor supervision needed)

Starting position

As in the main exercise.

Exercise

Inhale – push the body upwards and extend the spine (A, *see* opposite).
Exhale – release the hands to rock forwards onto the pelvis (B).
Inhale – catch the body with the hands on the mat (C).

Ending

Inhale – push the body upwards to extend spine.
Exhale – lower the body down towards the floor.

12 Shell stretch

This is a spine release exercise to be done after exercises executed in the prone position.

Starting position

Kneel down, legs slightly apart, feet together.

Exercise

Bend forward and stretch the arms in front of the head, with the forehead and palms of the hands on the floor. Breathe into the back when inhaling. Feel your tailbone weighted down to the floor. Feel the body relax into the position when exhaling. Stay in this relaxed pose for 10 to 15 seconds.

Muscular emphasis

Muscle release along the spine

Note:

- Individuals with limited knee flexion or uncomfortable hips should place one or two cushions on the back of the calves to release tension (i.e. sit on the cushion placed on the back of the legs).
- Alternatively, do the exercise sitting on a seat, hugging the knees, with rounded spine.

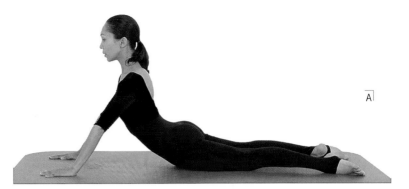

A

The advanced swan

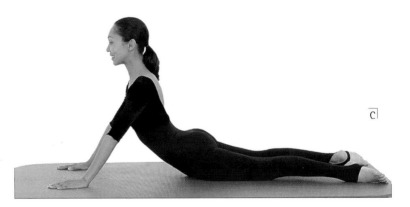

B

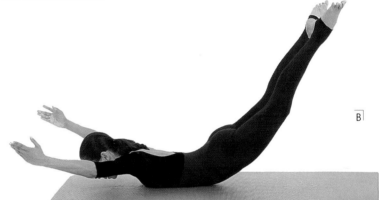

C

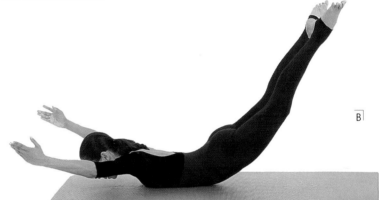

Shell stretch

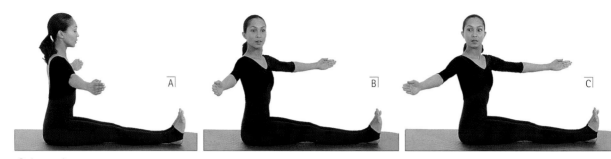

Spine twist

Spine twist

10 repetitions, alternating sides
Loosens the spine.
Increases hip and waist flexibility.

Starting position

Sit tall on the mat, with neutral spine, legs extended together in front, feet dorsi-flexed. Lift arms at your sides just below shoulder level, palms of the hands facing forwards (A).

Exercise

Inhale – three breaths to rotate the spine three times, turning from the waist to the right (one breath with every rotation – B, C, D). Lengthen the spine with each rotation. Turn the palm of the right hand backwards towards the spine on the third rotation (D). Look back at the right hand and feel the front shoulder opening.

Exhale – lengthen and grow even taller through the base of the spine, returning to the starting position (E). Repeat the exercise to the other side.

Visualization

Sitting on a bed of nails.

Muscular emphasis

Transversus abdominis; obliques; Erector spinae; multifidi

Note:

- If you tend to lift the shoulders reverse the breathing (i.e. use three short exhalations for each rotation rather than three short inhalations).
- If you have a tight lower back, tight hamstrings and/or hip flexors, sit on a pillow with your legs crossed.
- Keep both hips facing squarely to the front.

Side series

Strengthens and tones inner thighs, outer thighs and buttocks.

Starting position

Lie on your side, with your lower arm lengthened along the mat and your top hand on the mat to balance. The pelvis should be in neutral, and the legs straight under the pelvis (A).

Note:

- A cushion placed between the head and arm may be used to support the head.
- Avoid taking the legs behind the pelvis, which causes the lower back to arch.

EXERCISE A:

8–10 repetitions

Inhale – lengthen and lift the top leg

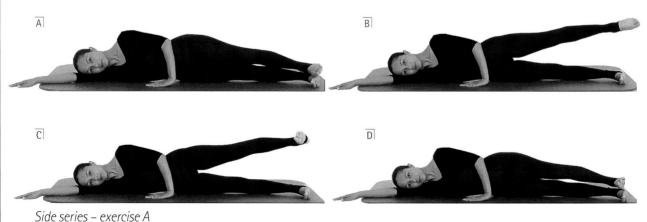

Side series – exercise A

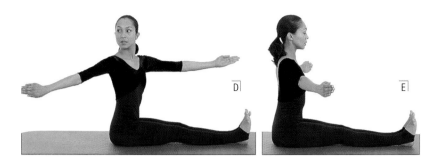

Exercise

Inhale – trace half a circle with your foot (B).

Exhale – complete the circle (C).

Visualization

The toe/heel is a pencil drawing a circle.

Muscular emphasis

Abdominals; adductors; abductors; gluteus muscles

Note:

- The working foot may be extended, pointed or dorsi-flexed.
- Leg length, not height, is important.
- Avoid shoulder tension.
- Ensure pelvic stability throughout.
- Support torso and lift bottom rib off the mat.

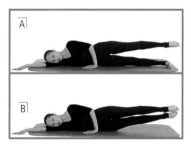

Side series – exercise B

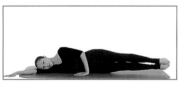

Side series – exercise C

---

to hip height, with foot pointed (B). Exhale – dorsi-flex the foot (C) and lengthen the leg out of the hip socket as you lower it (D).

Visualization

Squeeze and flatten a soft ball between the thighs when lowering the leg.

Muscular emphasis

Abdominals; hip abductors (outside of the hip)

EXERCISE B:

8–10 repetitions

Inhale – lengthen and extend the upper leg to hip height (A).

Exhale – lift the extended lower leg to meet the top leg (B) and press the bottom leg down with the top leg.

Visualization

Squeeze to flatten a soft ball under the legs as both legs lower.

Muscular emphasis

Lower leg adductors; upper leg adductors and abductors

EXERCISE C:

8–10 repetitions

Inhale.

Exhale – extend and lift both legs together into the air.

Inhale – lengthen and lower the legs with resistance.

Visualization

Think of the legs as a lever.

Muscular emphasis

Abdominals; lower leg adductors; upper leg adductors and abductors

EXERCISE D:

8 ankle circles one way, 8 in reverse

Preparation

Inhale.

Exhale – extend and lift the upper leg to hip height (A).

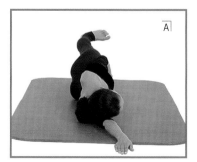

Side series – exercise D

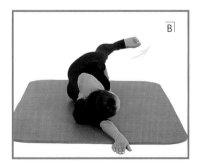

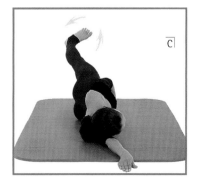

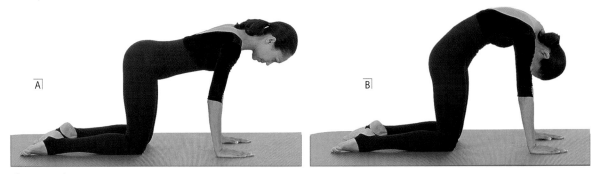

Cat stretch

15 Cat stretch

3–5 repetitions

Increases flexion and mobility of the spine.

Starting position

Kneel on all fours on the mat, making sure that you keep your head in line with the neutral spine (A).

Exercise

Inhale – flex the spine, moving the tailbone and crown of the head towards the floor (B).

Exhale – lengthen the spine back to neutral (A).

Visualization

Angry cat – spinal flexion.

Muscular emphasis

Abdominals; Erector spinae; multifidi

Note:

• Avoid 'winging' (pressing shoulder blades together) on the spine extension.

• Do not hyper-extend the elbows.

16 Swimming

5 sets

(Five short inhalations, five short exhalations = one set; same breathing pattern as for 'the hundred')

Improves co-ordination.

Starting position

Lie on your stomach, arms extended in front, shoulder-distance apart, legs lengthened along the mat, hip-distance apart (A).

Inhale.

Exhale – lift arms and legs just off the mat.

Exercise

Inhale – lift and lower arms and legs contra-laterally (opposite arms to legs as if swimming) for five counts = five short inhalations or 'sniffs' (B).

Exhale – lift and lower arms and legs contra-laterally for five short exhalations (B).

Ending

Inhale – remain still.

Exhale – lower arms and legs.

Visualization

Splashing water with straight limbs.

Muscular emphasis

Deltoids; obliques; Latissimus dorsi; gluteus muscles; Transversus abdominis; multifidi; Erector spinae

PREPARATORY EXERCISE A:

5 repetitions

Work only the legs as a separate exercise, applying the same preparation, breathing pattern and ending as in the main exercise.

PREPARATORY EXERCISE B:

5 repetitions

Work only the arms as a separate exercise, applying the same preparation, breathing pattern and ending as in the main exercise.

Note:

• Avoid lumbar strain and shoulder elevation.

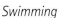

Swimming

- Do not hold your breath.
- Maintain leg extension from the hips.
- Extend arms and legs just off the mat.

17 The seal

10 repetitions
Improves balance.
Improves co-ordination.

Starting position

Sit on the mat, spine flexed, soles of the feet together, knees bent. Extend hands through the centre of your legs to hold the outside of the ankles. Raise the feet off the mat to balance just off the sitting bones (A).

Exercise

Inhale – rock backwards then clap the soles of the feet together three times (B). Do not rock onto the cervical (neck) area.

Exhale – rock forwards to balance in the starting position (A) and clap the soles of the feet together three times.

Visualization

Base of a rocking horse.

Muscular emphasis

Abdominals; external rotators of the hip; shoulder girdle stabilizers

Note:

- Do not lose the C-curve.
- Avoid rolling onto the cervical spine.

PREPARATORY EXERCISE:

Omit clapping until balance is established.

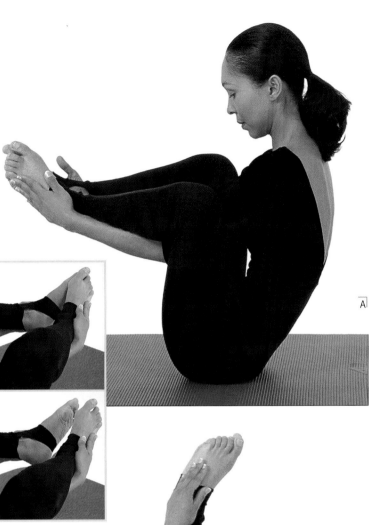

A

Above **Close-up of clapping feet, which helps to work the peronial muscles on the outside of the lower leg.**

B

The seal

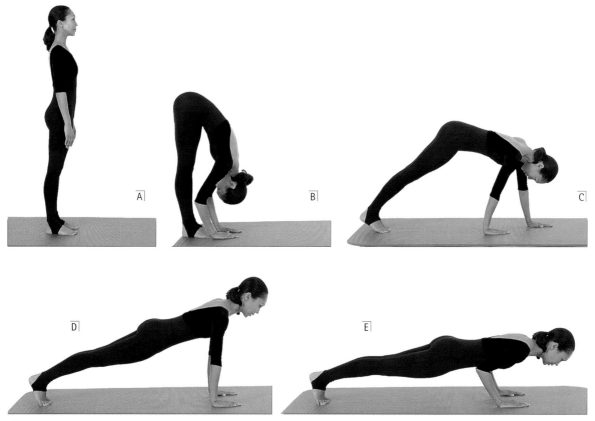

Press-ups

18 Press-ups

3–5 repetitions

A strengthening exercise.

Starting position

Stand tall at the end of the mat with feet hip-width apart (A).

Exercise

Inhale.

Exhale – curl down towards the floor, rolling down one vertebra at a time (B). Inhale (B).

Exhale – take four walks forward with hands along the floor (C) to establish the push-up position (D). Inhale – take three short inhalations or sniffs. With each sniff, bend your elbows a little more (E) in order to lower your body towards the mat (sniff, sniff, sniff = lower, lower, lower).

Exhale – three short exhalations, each time extending the elbows a little more into a push-up (exhale, exhale, exhale = extend, extend, extend (D)).

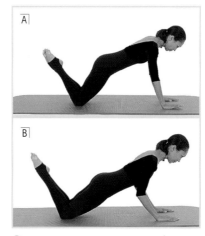

Press ups - preparatory exercise

Inhale – walk your hands backwards (C) to the end of the mat (B).

Exhale – roll up, one vertebra at a time, back to a standing position (A).

Visualization

Sink sink sink; grow grow grow.

Muscular emphasis

Abdominals; hip adductors; hamstrings; gluteus muscles; Serratus anterior (upper ribs at side of the chest); lower trapezius; biceps; triceps

Note:

• Keep bottom rib pulled inwards.

PREPARATORY EXERCISE:

10 repetitions

Starting position

Kneel down with hands hip-width apart on the mat, feet lifted into the air (A).

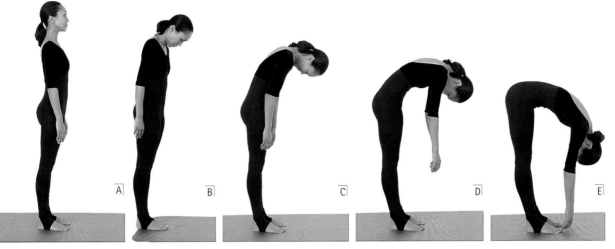

Roll down

Exercise

As for the main exercise:

Inhale – three sniffs to bend elbows, lowering the torso towards the mat with each sniff (B).

Exhale – three exhalations to extend the elbows, lifting the torso with each exhalation (A).

Note:

- Avoid 'winging' the shoulder blades.
- Do not drop the pelvis too low or lift it too high in the push-up position: aim for a straight line from head to toe.

19 Roll down

3–5 repetitions

This is a good end-of-session exercise that helps with spine articulation.

Starting position

Stand with your back against a wall, feet parallel and hip-width apart (A). Feet should be the length of your own foot away from wall. Lengthen upwards through the tips of your ears to avoid tilting your head backwards.

Exercise

Inhale – to 'nod' (B)'

Exhale – starting with the cervical spine (neck), roll the spine down towards the floor, flexing one vertebra at a time (C, D, E).

Inhale – retain the full forward bend (E).

Exhale – starting with the lower back, roll back to the starting position, one vertebra at a time (D, C, B, A).

Visualization

Peel the spine off the wall, then glue the spine back onto the wall.

Muscular emphasis

Abdominals; multifidi; Erector spinae; Quadratus lumborum; Latissimus dorsi; trapezius

Note:

- Roll down only as far as you can without forcing it.
- Take your mind into your spine.
- The exercise is only effective when executed slowly.
- Avoid tilting the head back.

20 Meditation

Heightens awareness of the senses.
Exercises facial muscles.

Starting position

Lie on your back on the mat, feet flat, knees bent, legs hip-width apart, arms at your sides, eyes closed, mouth open, jaw dropped and tongue towards the back of your throat.

Exercise

Meditate the following points:

1. Feel the weight of your body as it weighs heavily down into the mat. Meditate 30 seconds to one minute.
2. Obliterate all thoughts entering your mind and listen to every sound around you. Meditate 30 seconds to one minute.
3. Feel your clothes on your body. Meditate 30 seconds to one minute.
4. Sense the air around you. Meditate 30 seconds to one minute.
5. Slowly lift and lower one finger at a time, starting with the baby fingers. Wait for five seconds after lifting each one.
6. Scrunch the hands into fists, then relax. Wait 10 seconds.
7. Scrunch the toes, then relax. Wait 10 seconds.
8. Scrunch the face, then relax. Wait 10 seconds.
9. Open eyes gently and recover to greet the rest of your day.

THE MORE ADVANCED ROUTINE

ONCE the step-by-step routine has been mastered, the more challenging advanced routine will provide an added incentive to your workout. These exercises are additions to the step-by-step routine and should only be attempted once the basics are secure.

1
Teaser

5 repetitions
(Not recommended for those with lower back problems)
Challenges abdominal strength. Lengthens the spine.

Starting position

Lie on your back, spine imprinted throughout. Reach arms back over the head. Extend legs together in the air, as low as possible (A).

Exercise

Inhale – raise the arms (B) and lift the torso. Reach arms and feet towards each other to form a 'V' (C).
Exhale – roll back down to the mat away from legs, keeping arms next to the ears and legs in the air (D).

Ending

Exhale – lower legs, one at a time.

Visualization

A balanced 'V' shape.

Muscular emphasis

Abdominals; hip flexors; shoulder girdle stabilizers

Note:

- Aim to roll down through each vertebra.
- Retain abdominal contraction.
- Avoid lifting shoulders.

PREPARATORY EXERCISE A:

5 repetitions
This is a good exercise to use before 'the hundred' in the step-by-step routine.

Starting position

Lie on your back on the mat with

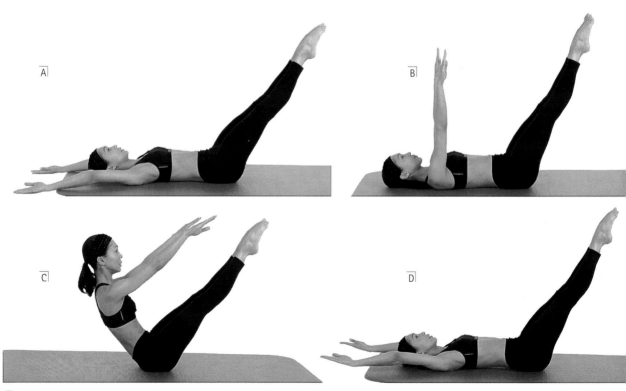

A | B | C | D

Teaser

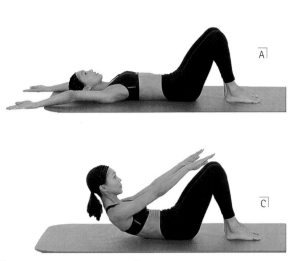

Teaser – preparatory exercise

your feet hip-width apart, knees bent, arms extended backwards on the mat, and palms facing the ceiling (A).

Exercise

Inhale – lift arms next past the ears and 'nod' (B).

Exhale – flex the spine and roll up, taking arms forward just above shoulder level (C).

Inhale – lift arms to the ears (D).

Exhale – roll back down to the starting position (A).

PREPARATORY EXERCISE B:

5 repetitions

As in Preparatory Exercise A, but with the legs together in the air and knees flexed above the hips.

2 Open leg rocker

10 repetitions

Builds abdominal control.

Starting position

Sit just off the sitting bones in a slight backward pelvic tilt. Lengthen the thoracic spine and extend the legs just wider than the shoulders. Hold the front of your ankles or sides of your legs with your hands (A).

Exercise

Inhale – using the C-curve, roll backwards onto the mat as shown (B, C).

Exhale – roll back up to balance. Lengthen through the mid-back, opening and lifting the chest without 'popping' the ribcage (A).

Visualization

An archer's bow.

Muscular emphasis

Abdominals; Erector spinae; multifidi; hamstrings; gluteus muscles; hip flexors; shoulder girdle stabilizers

Note:

- Lead the movement with the lower back.
- Do not arch the lower back.
- Avoid rolling into the cervical spine (neck area).

PREPARATORY EXERCISE:

10 repetitions

As in the main exercise but bend the knees.

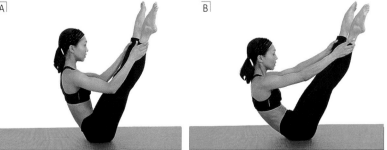

Open leg rocker

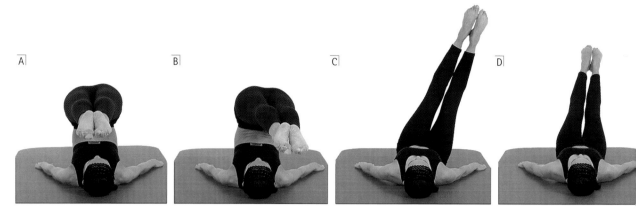

Corkscrew

3 Corkscrew

3–6 repetitions either side, alternating
Builds strength.
Improves control.

Starting position

Lie on your back on the mat, legs together in the air, arms at your sides, spine imprinted.

Preparation

Inhale.

Exhale – roll the spine off the mat and take your legs overhead until they are parallel to the floor (A).

Exercise

Inhale – pull toes towards right ear (B).
Exhale – take the feet down the right side of the spine as you roll down through the spine onto the mat (C, D). Take the feet up left side of spine to roll the spine up off the mat (E).

Inhale – centre the legs parallel to the floor (A).
Repeat on the other side.

Visualization

A 'U' shape.

Muscular emphasis

Abdominals, especially obliques; shoulder girdle stabilizers; hamstrings; hip flexors

Note:

- Do not arch your back.
- Retain ribcage placement.
- Avoid rolling into the cervical spine (neck area).

PREPARATORY EXERCISE:

3–6 repetitions

Starting position

Lean back off the sitting bones, supporting the torso with the elbows at your sides and your

legs extended together in the air.

Exercise

Inhale – pull the toes of both feet together towards the right ear.
Exhale – lower the legs down the right side of the spine, then lift them up the left side of the spine.
Repeat on the other side.

Visualization

A small 'U' shape.

4 Full swan dive:

10 repetitions (forward and back = one repetition)
Strengthens back, neck and shoulders.

Starting position

Lie on your stomach on the mat, hands next to your shoulders, legs slightly apart and turned outwards.

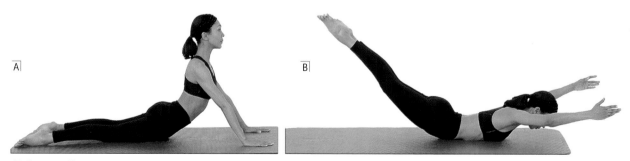

Full swan dive

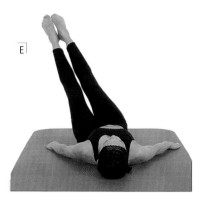

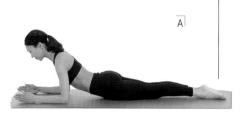

Single leg kick

6–10 repetitions per leg, alternating
(Supervision needed; avoid if you have
knee problems)

Starting position

Lie on your stomach on the mat,
supporting the torso on bent elbows,
with palms of your hands facing one
another. The head should follow the
line of the spine, the legs are
together and the pelvis in a
backward tilt (A).

Exercise

Inhale.

Exhale – bend one knee and
tap/pulse the foot towards the
buttocks, first with a pointed toe (B),
then with a dorsi-flexed foot (C).
Inhale – extend the leg back to the
starting position (D).
Repeat with the other leg.

Muscular emphasis

Abdominals; gluteus muscles;
hamstrings; shoulder girdle stabilizers

Note:

- Do not arch your back.
- Retain abdominal contraction and
  accurate ribcage placement.
- Avoid shoulder tension and/or
  'winging' the shoulders.

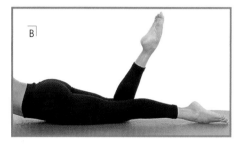

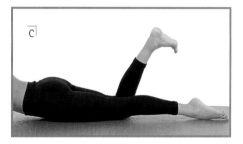

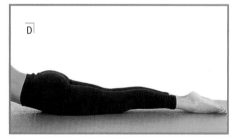

Single leg kick

Exercise

Inhale – push up with your hands
and arms, lengthening the spine (A).
Exhale – lift the arms off the mat
(next to the ears) and rock forward
onto the ribcage, lifting the extended
legs behind you (B, C).
Inhale – rock back onto the pelvis
(D). Rock 10 times, then end.

Ending

Inhale – catch the torso with the
hands.
Exhale – lower the torso back to the
mat.

Visualization

A rocking banana.

(For muscular emphasis and preparatory exercise, *see* 'the swan', page 62)

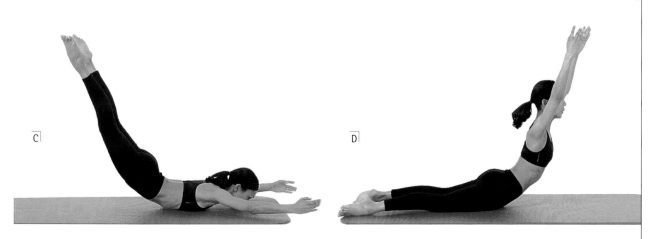

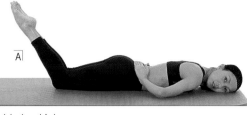

Double leg kick

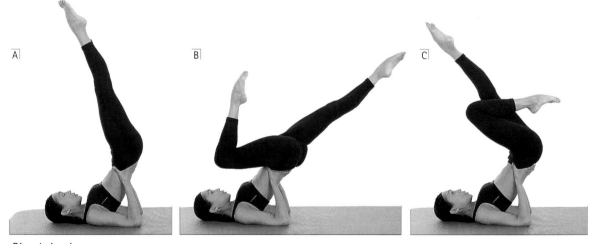

Double leg kick

3–5 repetitions each side, alternating
(Supervision needed; avoid if you have
lower back or knee problems)
Stretches the lower back.

Starting position

Lie on your stomach with legs
together, head turned to one side
and hands behind your back (A).

Exercise

Inhale.

Exhale – bend both knees to tap/pulse
feet three times towards the buttocks
– three short exhalations (B).

Inhale – extend the legs, slightly turned
out. Lengthen and extend the spine as
the arms extend at your sides and the
upper torso lifts off the mat (C).

Exhale – lower the torso to the mat
and return to starting position. Turn
your head to the other side and
repeat the exercise.

Visualization

Lengthen like a torpedo on
inhalation.

Muscular emphasis

Abdominals; hamstrings; lower
gluteus muscles; Erector spinae;
multifidi; Latissimus dorsi; shoulder
girdle stabilizers

Note:

- Avoid arching the back.
- Do not let the tailbone ride up
  and down.
- Retain shoulder blade stabilization.

Bicycle in the air

20 repetitions, each direction
(To be avoided by those with lower
back or neck problems)
Builds strength and improves balance,
control and co-ordination.

Starting position

Shoulder-stand on the mat, with
hands supporting the back, legs
parallel in the air (A).

Exercise

Inhale – extend one leg and bend
the other leg at the knee to create a
cycling motion (B).

Bicycle in air

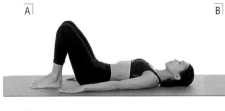

A

B

C

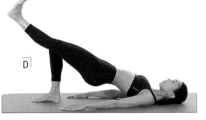

D

Shoulder bridge

Exhale – bend the knee of the extended leg and extend the other leg (C).
Reverse direction after 20 repetitions.

Visualization
Cycling action.

Muscular emphasis
Hamstrings; gluteus muscles; abdominals; Quadratus lumborum

Note:
- Avoid over-extending the lumbar spine.
- Avoid neck pressure.

8 Shoulder bridge

3 repetitions each side
(Supervision needed; avoid if you have lower back or neck problems, tennis elbow or carpal tunnel syndrome)
Tests core stability and strength.

Starting position
Lie on your back on the mat, legs hip-width apart, knees flexed, soles of the feet on the mat, arms at your sides (A).

Preparation
Inhale.
Exhale – lift the pelvis off the mat, maintaining a neutral spine (B).

Exercise
Inhale – bend the left knee towards the chest.
Exhale – extend left leg in the air (C).
Inhale – dorsi-flex the left foot as the left leg lowers towards the supporting knee (D).
Exhale – again lift left leg up towards the ceiling and point the foot (C).
Lower and lift the leg twice more.
Inhale – place left foot back on mat.
Exhale – lift the right leg up to the ceiling.
Repeat the exercise with right leg.

Ending
Inhale – lower the suspended leg (B).
Exhale – lower the pelvis, replacing the hips on the mat (A).

Visualization
A bridge.

Muscular emphasis
Hamstrings; gluteus muscles; hip flexors; abdominals

Note:
- Avoid neck pressure or over-extending the lumbar spine.
- Retain hamstring connection.
- Avoid pressing down on your wrists or elbows.

9 Pleadings

6–8 repetitions
Improves balance, control and co-ordination.

Starting position
Lie on your back, legs together, knees flexed, arms at your sides (A).

Exercise
Inhale.
Exhale – roll onto the left side and balance on your left hip. Rotate the upper torso to the right, with arms and shoulders in an oblique line to the right, arms just below shoulder level and palms facing the ceiling. Your eye line should be towards your hands (B). Sustain the pose to the end of the exhalation.
Inhale – roll down to the mat and return to the starting position.
Repeat on the other side.

Visualization
Pleading pose.

Muscular emphasis
Abdominals, especially obliques; hip flexors; shoulder girdle stabilizers

Note:
- Avoid upper body tension.
- Balance on the side of the hip.

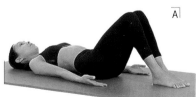

A

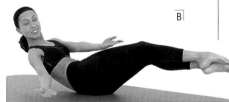

B

Pleadings

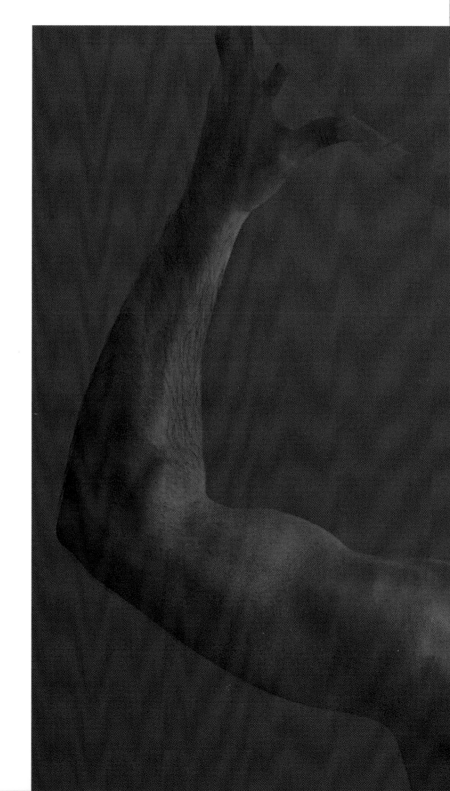

Ten minutes a day

Tea-break Pilates

Additional stretches

Medical conditions

ADDITIONAL
ROUTINES

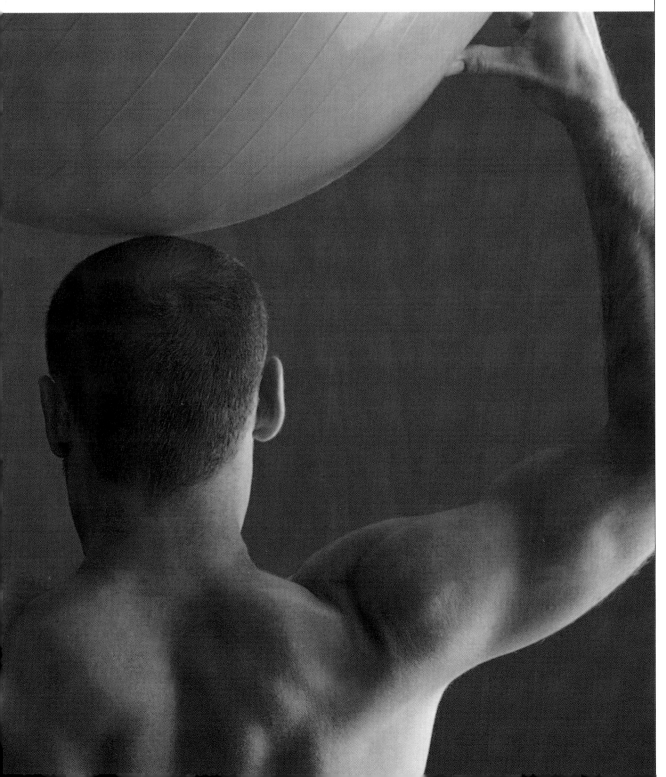

TEN MINUTES A DAY

THIS short, ten-minute routine of simple, yet effective, exercises can be used on days when you do not do the full, step-by-step session.

1 Pelvic tilt

6–10 repetitions
Mobilizes the spine.

Starting position

Lie on your back with legs hip-width apart, knees flexed, soles of the feet on the mat, arms at your sides and your pelvis in the neutral position (A).

Exercise

Inhale.

Exhale – tilt the pelvis backwards so the lower back flattens onto the mat. Roll up through the spine, one vertebra at a time, to the end of the thoracic spine or upper back (B). Inhale – sustain the position with your hips in the air (B).

Exhale – roll down, one vertebra at a time, back to the starting position.

Muscular emphasis

Abdominals; multifidi; Erector spinae

Note:

● Avoid rolling into the cervical spine (neck area).

PELVIC TILT VARIATION A:

6–10 repetitions

As in the main exercise, but squeezing a pillow between the knees to use the inner thigh muscles.

PELVIC TILT VARIATION B:

6–10 repetitions

As in the main exercise, but with one knee crossed over the other to roll up on one supporting leg. This works the hamstrings and lower gluteus muscles even more.

2 Abdominal preparation

8–10 repetitions
Builds abdominal strength.

Starting position

Lie on your back with legs hip-width apart, knees flexed, soles of the feet on the mat, arms at your sides and pelvis in the neutral position (A).

Exercise

Inhale – to 'nod'.

Exhale – bend the upper body and slide the ribcage towards the pelvis, with your arms just off the mat (B). Inhale – hold the position.

Exhale – lower the upper body back to the starting position (A).

Muscular emphasis

Abdominals; shoulder girdle stabilizers

Note:

● For neck tension, place a towel under the head and lift the towel with the hands. Or place your hands under your head for support.

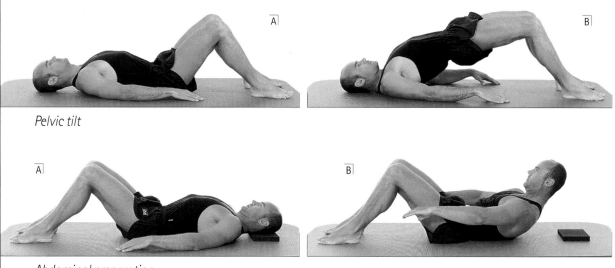

Pelvic tilt

Abdominal preparation

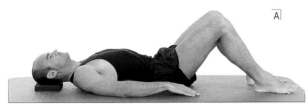

Knee lift

3
Knee lift

6 repetitions, alternate sides
(Recommended for beginners or those
with lower back problems)
Stabilizes the pelvis.

Starting position

Lie on your back, with legs hip-width
apart, knees bent, soles of the feet on
the mat, arms at your sides and neutral pelvis (A).

Exercise

Inhale.
Exhale – peel the left foot off the
floor, heel first, then the toes. Lift the
flexed left knee into the air until the

thigh is at 90 degrees to the floor (B).
Inhale – hold the position.
Exhale – lower the left knee back to
the starting position, placing the toes
down first, then the heel.
Repeat with the right leg.

Muscular emphasis

Abdominals; hip flexors; soleus and
gastrocnemius (calf muscles)

Note:

* Retain pelvic stability when lifting
  the legs.
* The pelvis and lower back should
  not move nor arch like the San
  Francisco bridge.

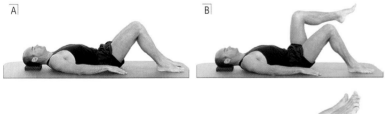

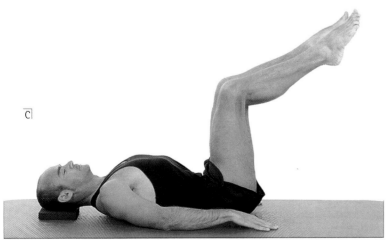

Knee lift - 'the bug'

4
Knee lift ('the bug')

4 repetitions
Establishes accurate use of
abdominals and spinal imprint.

Starting position

Lie on your back, with legs hip-width
apart, knees flexed, soles of the feet
on the mat, arms at your sides and
neutral spine (A).

Exercise

Inhale. Exhale – raise one bent knee
into the air (B).
Inhale. Exhale – imprint the spine,
then raise the other flexed knee into
the air (C).
Inhale. Exhale – lower the first leg
back to the starting position,
retaining the spinal imprint (B).
Inhale. Exhale – lower the other leg to
the starting position (A).
Repeat the sequence starting with the
other leg.

Visualization

A bug on its back.

Muscular emphasis

Abdominals; hip flexors; soleus and
gastrocnemius (calf muscles)

Note:

* To avoid injury, take care to retain
  pelvic stability and abdominal
  contraction when lifting the legs.
* Ensure that the pelvis and lower
  back do not move or arch like
  a bridge.

Side leg lifts

8–10 repetitions per level

Works the outer thighs.

Starting position

Lie on your side with legs extended together, lower arm lengthened along the mat, upper arm placed forward for balance (A). A cushion may be placed between the head and lower arm for head support. The spine should be neutral, lower ribs lifted off the mat, and legs slightly forward to prevent arching the lower back.

First level: lift the top leg 10cm (4in) away from the bottom leg, then lower it again (B).

Second level: lift the top leg 20cm (8in) away from the bottom leg (A). Lower it by about 10cm (4in), i.e. the leg remains suspended (B).

Third level: lift the top leg 30cm (12in) away from the bottom leg (A). Lower it by about 10cm (4in), i.e. the leg remains suspended, slightly higher this time.

Exercise, with breathing

Join all three levels together, breathing as described

First level:

Inhale – lift the top leg 10cm (4in)

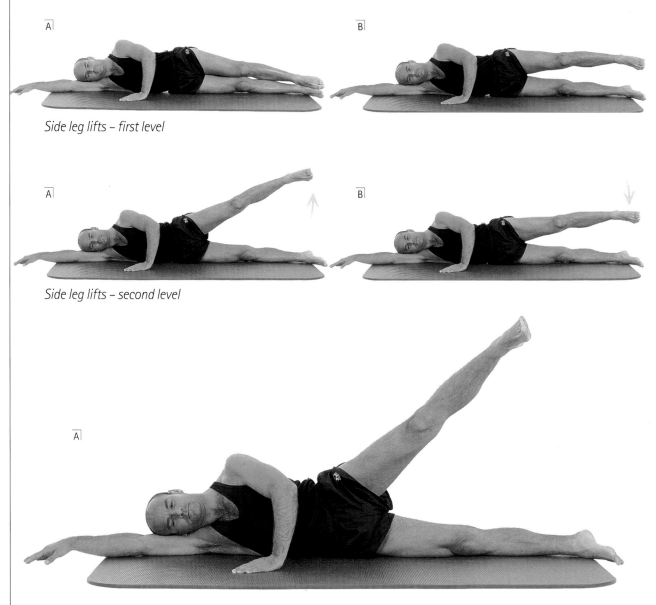

A

B

Side leg lifts – first level

A

B

Side leg lifts – second level

A

Side leg lifts – third level

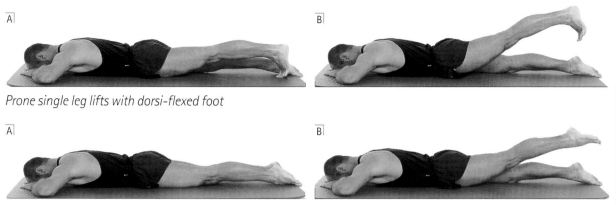

Prone single leg lifts with dorsi-flexed foot

Prone single leg lifts with extended foot

away from the bottom leg (B).
Exhale – lower the top leg, with
resistance, to the bottom leg (A).

Second level:

Inhale – lift the top leg 20cm (8in)
away from the bottom leg (A).
Exhale – lower the leg only 10cm
(4in) so it remains suspended (B).

Third level:

Inhale – starting from the second
level's suspended position, lift the top
leg 30cm (12in) away from the
bottom leg (A).

Exhale – lower the leg only 10cm
(4in) so that it remains suspended.

Ending

Inhale – pause in the air.
Exhale – lower the leg back to the
starting position.

Visualization

A lever at different levels.

Muscular emphasis

Abductors (outer thigh muscles);
adductors (inner thigh muscles)

Note:

• Retain length of the leg throughout.
• Drop the foot down from the ankle
  to create extra weight.
• Apply resistance when lowering.

Exhale – lower the extended leg
again to the mat (A).
Repeat with the other leg.

Visualization

A lever.

Muscular emphasis

Abdominals; lower gluteus muscles;
hip extensors (hamstrings)

Note:

• Both hips should remain on the
  floor throughout.
• Aim to extend the leg from the hip.
• Avoid lifting the tailbone.

Prone single leg lifts

10 repetitions, alternating legs
*(May be executed with a dorsi-flexed
or extended foot)*
Tones the buttocks.

Starting position

Lie on your stomach on the mat, with
lengthened legs and forehead resting
on your hands between the thumbs
and pointers (A). Palms to the floor,
touch thumb to thumb and pointer to
pointer to form a diamond shape.

Exercise

Inhale – lift one extended leg (B).

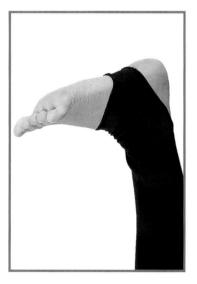

Above **Close-up of prone single leg
lifts showing dorsi-flexion.**

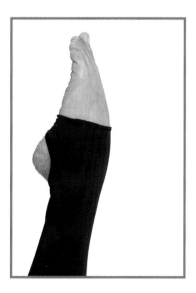

Above **Close-up of prone single leg
lifts showing foot extension.**

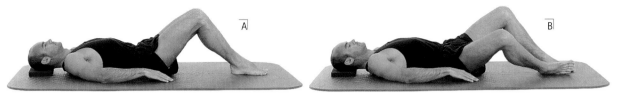

Side centre side

7 Side centre side

10 repetitions, each leg
Builds control.
Strengthens abdominal muscles.
Hip muscles work smoothly together in a balanced manner.

Starting position
Lie on your back, with legs together, knees flexed, soles of the feet on the mat, arms at your sides and spine neutral (A).

Exercise
Inhale.
Exhale – open the right knee to the side with a smooth, continuous movement (B).
Inhale.
Exhale – return to the starting position with a controlled, smooth and continuous movement (A).
Repeat with the left knee.

Visualization
A fan opening.

Muscular emphasis
Abdominals; hip flexors; hip adductors – especially to prevent legs from 'flopping' out to the side

Note:
• Retain accurate pelvic placement – do not let hips sway from side to side.

8 Hip rolls

10 repetitions, alternate sides
Helps to release the lower back.

Starting position
Lie on your back, with legs together, knees flexed, soles of the feet on the mat, arms at your sides and spine neutral (A).

Exercise
Inhale.
Exhale – roll the knees to the side, keeping the buttocks and shoulders on the mat (B).
Inhale.
Exhale – return to the starting position (A).
Repeat on the other side.

Muscular emphasis
Abdominals (especially obliques); adductors; Lattissimus dorsi

Note:
• Roll to the side without twisting at the waist or lifting your shoulders off the mat.

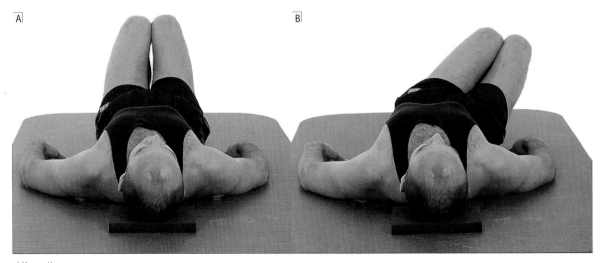

Hip rolls

TEA-BREAK PILATES

NECK and shoulder tension are common problems caused by stress and by sitting at a desk with bad posture for many hours. Poor posture causes the upper trapezius muscle to become shortened and contracted, moving the shoulders slightly up and forward.

To release the tension:
- Sit or stand tall.
- Pull shoulder blades down towards the hips.
- Open the pectoral muscles to open your chest without the ribcage 'popping' or the shoulder blades 'winging'.

The following exercises, designed to release tension and energize the body, can be performed during a tea break or lunch break from work.

1 Just breathe

10 repetitions

Starting position
Sit tall on a chair without arching the back.

Exercise
Place your hands on your ribcage (A). Apply the Pilates breathing technique as follows.
Inhale – fill the lungs with oxygen and feel the ribcage expanding sideways (B).
Exhale – contract the abdominals and flatten the belly towards the spine (A).

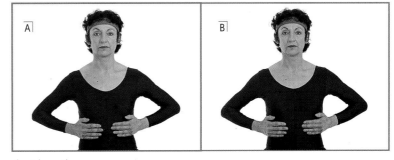

Just breathe

2 Alphabet

Alleviates neck tension.

Starting position
Sit tall, with head erect.

Exercise
Trace the letters of the alphabet with your nose (A–E, etc).

Visualization
The point of your nose is a pencil.

Muscular emphasis
Splenius muscles (at the back of the neck); sternocleidomastoid muscle (at the sides of the neck); deep neck flexors

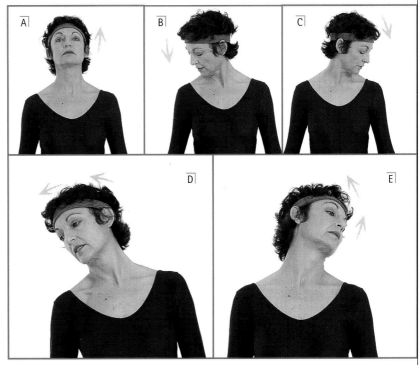

Alphabet

3 Inclined neck stretch

6 repetitions, alternating sides
Releases neck and upper body tension.

Starting position

Sit tall, arms at your sides, head erect.

Exercise

Inhale – fold the right hand over the top of the head towards the left ear (A). Exhale – gently pull the head towards the right (B). Hold for eight seconds. Repeat on the other side.

Muscular emphasis

Upper trapezius, splenius muscles (back of the neck); abdominals; sternocleidomastoid (sides of the neck)

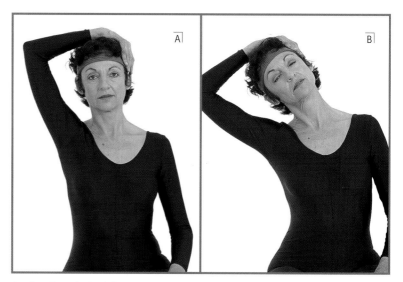

Inclined neck stretch

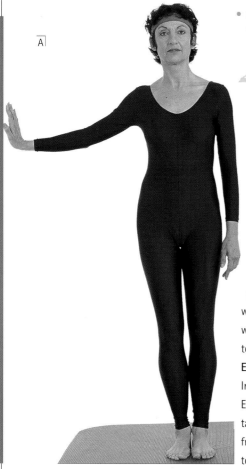

Neural arm exercises

Note:

- Retain eye focus to the front.
- Avoid slightly turning the head or 'jutting' the chin forward.

4 Neural arm exercises

(Repeat only once in each position)
Releases upper body tension.
There are three different hand positions:

HAND POSITION A:

Starting position

Stand sideways next to a wall. With the arm fully stretched, extend the wrist to place the palm of the hand flat against the wall just below shoulder height, with fingers spread and extended towards the ceiling (A).

Exercise

Inhale.
Exhale – lean slightly forwards and take three to four small steps away from the palm, which remains glued to the wall. Feel the front of the shoulder and pectorals opening.

Inhale.
Exhale – take three to four small steps back to the starting position.

HAND POSITION B:

(Hand laterally rotated)

Starting position

As in position A, but now spread

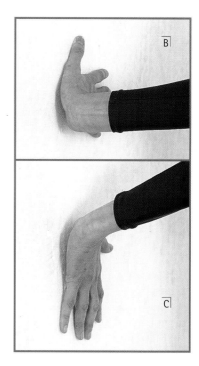

and extend the fingers so that they point towards the back (B).

Exercise

As in hand position A.

HAND POSITION C:

(Hand medially rotated)

Starting position

As in hand position A, but now spread and extend the fingers downward to the floor (C).

Exercise

As in hand position A.

Muscular emphasis

Abdominals; deltoids; trapezius; shoulder girdle stabilizers

Note:

- Avoid taking the arm too high, causing the shoulder to lift.

5 Elevation and depression

A daily exercise for those suffering from neck and upper body tension (*see* 'warm-up exercises' on page 44).

6 Sliding down the wall

10 repetitions

Works knees and thighs.

Starting position

Stand with your back against the wall, feet parallel and hip-width apart and neutral pelvis (A).

Exercise

Inhale.

Exhale – bend the knees to slide the thoracic (upper back) and lumbar (lower back) spine down the wall (B).

Inhale – extend the legs to slide back to the starting position (A).

Visualization

As if sitting down then change your mind to stand up.

Muscular emphasis

Quadriceps; hamstrings; shoulder girdle stabilizers; abdominals; deep neck flexors

Note:

- Avoid 'jamming' the head against the wall in the start/end position.
- Firmly retain upper body and shoulder girdle placement.

7 Roll down

10 repetitions

For this exercise, see the 'step-by-step' section on page 69.

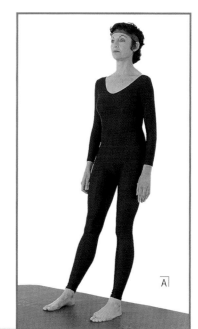

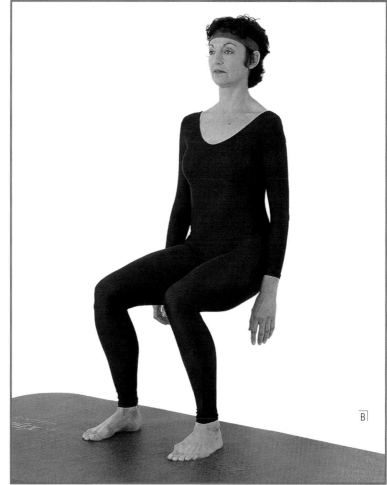

Sliding down the wall

ADDITIONAL STRETCHES

1 Simple rises

10 repetitions

Centres the body through accurate leg and foot alignment.

Starting position

Stand upright with good postural alignment, holding onto the back of a chair with both hands (A).

Exercise

Inhale – rise through the feet onto the balls of the feet for three counts, feeling the crown of the head is the highest point (B).

Exhale – lower through the feet for three counts.

('Up two three, down two three'.)

Visualization

Rise up through the tips of your ears.

Muscular emphasis

Abdominals; soleus and gastrocnemius (calf muscles);

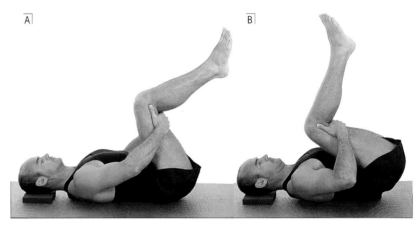

Lower back release

quadriceps; intrinsic muscles (in the foot)

Note:

- Retain accurate alignment of the leg and foot (see page 23).
- Avoid rolling the feet inwards or outwards.

2 Lower back release

10 repetitions

Stretches and releases tension in the lower back.

Starting position

Lie on your back, imprint the spine and bend knees towards your chest. Hold onto the back of the knees with your hands (A).

Exercise

Inhale.

Exhale – gently pull the knees towards the chest (B).

Inhale – release the legs.

3 Shoulder stretch

6 repetitions

Works the back of the shoulders. (Those with hip problems should sit cross-legged on a cushion.)

Starting position

Sit upright on a cushion placed between the back of the calves and the buttocks, arms at your sides and palms facing forward (A).

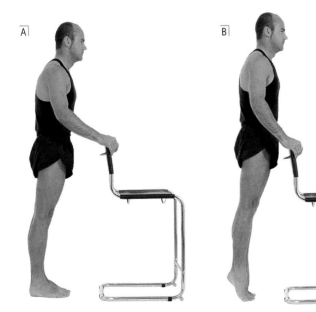

Simple rises

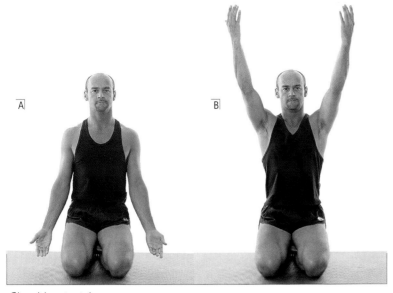

Shoulder stretch

Exercise

Inhale – lift arms overhead, retaining scapular and shoulder girdle placement.

Exhale – pull arms backwards while pulling the ribcage forward (B). The movement is minimal and comes from within.

Inhale – hold.

Exhale – repeat as for the previous exhalation (B).

Visualization

Strive to reach the palms of the hands towards the wall behind you without moving your shoulders.

Muscular emphasis

Abdominals; shoulder girdle stabilizers; trapezius; pectorals; anterior (front) deltoid

4 Hamstring stretch

4 repetitions

Starting position

Crouch on all fours, arms shoulder-width apart. Keep your heels up, balancing on the balls of the feet (A).

Exercise

Inhale.

Exhale – push up to extend the elbows and legs, and lower the heels to touch the mat, keeping all 10 fingers firmly down (B). The sitting bones should be the highest point in the air. Move the chest towards the thighs and retain lengthened thighs while the sitting bones move upward. Heels remain on the floor.

Inhale and exhale, retaining the position and feeling the stretch (B). Return to starting position.

Visualization

An upside down 'V' shape.

Muscular emphasis

Hamstrings; shoulder girdle stabilizers; abdominals; calf muscles; Erector spinae

Note:

- Do not lift shoulders towards ears.
- Retain the line of the upper spine – do not look up.

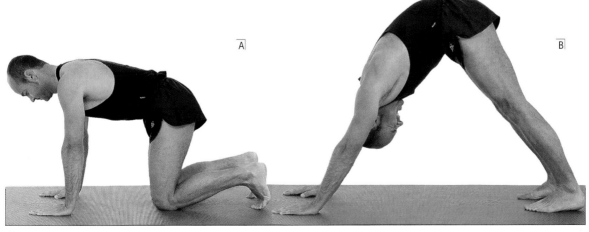

Hamstring stretch

MEDICAL CONDITIONS

IT is said that, through his exercises, Joseph Pilates was one of the first physiotherapists. Today, physiotherapists, chiropractors and medical doctors familiar with the Pilates strengthening programme are supportive of its benefits. Redressing muscle imbalances and strengthening the muscles correctly helps many people suffering from osteoarthritis, osteoporosis, shoulder and knee problems, headaches, stress, sciatica, and hip and back problems.

Pilates is not, however, a 'quick fix'. Instead, it should be used on a daily basis as a maintenance programme.

This section suggests some exercises for people suffering from:

1 Osteoarthritis of the hip
2 Tendonitis
3 Headaches
4 Back problems and sciatica
5 Shoulder conditions
6 Carpal tunnel syndrome
7 Knee problems
8 Ankle and foot problems

1 Osteoarthritis of the hip

It is vital for the hip to move through its full range of movement.

(a) Suggested exercises from the **warm-up and stretching** routines:
Easy hamstring stretch (page 49)
Easy groin stretch (page 47)
Easy hip stretch (page 47)
Easy hip flexor stretch (page 49)
(b) Suggested exercises from the **step-by-step** routine:
Leg circles (page 57)
Side series (page 64)
Swimming (page 66)
The seal (page 67)
Note:
• Take care to correct and improve postural alignment.

2 Tendonitis

Tendonitus caused by repetitive movement can occur in any part of the body. Take short breaks during repetitive work and move the sore joints through a range of movements specific to the affected area.

Qualified Pilates instructors can advise about exercises for specific problem areas.

3 Headaches

Headaches are often caused by tension created through emotional stress or bad posture. Releasing the upper trapezius muscle will provide relief. Do all the exercises from the **warm-up** routine (pages 44–46). Do all the exercises from **tea-break Pilates** (pages 83–85).

4 Back problems and sciatica

These exercises will help to relieve the pain. Take care not to strain the back or do too many repetitions.
(a) Suggested exercises from the **step-by-step** routine:
The hundred (page 54) – imprint spine
Single leg stretch (page 58) – imprint spine
Side to side obliques (page 59) – imprint spine
Diamond press (page 61)
Shell stretch (page 63)
Cat stretch (page 66)
Swimming (page 66)
Note:
• Take care to correct and improve postural alignment.
(b) Suggested exercises from the **ten minutes a day** routine:
Pelvic tilt (page 78)
Abdominal preparation (page 78)
Hip rolls (page 82)
(c) Suggested exercise from the **step-by-step** routine:

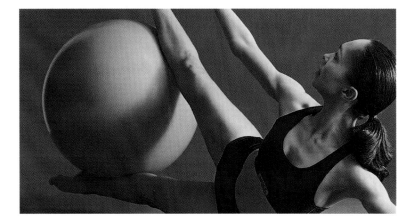

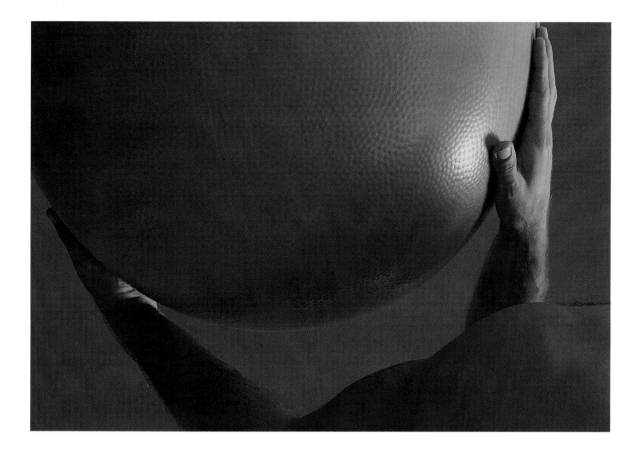

Roll down (page 69)

(d) Suggested exercise from **additional stretches:**

Lower back release (page 86)

Shoulder conditions

Suprispinatus tendonitis

Frozen shoulder

Rotator cuff muscle problems

Note:

- If pain worsens, stop the exercise immediately.
- Avoid excessive repetitions.

(a) Suggested exercises from the **warm-up** routine:

Elevation and depression (page 44)

Protraction and retraction (page 44)

Crossing elbows (page 44)

Elbow circles (page 45)

The dumb waiter (page 46)

(b) Suggested exercise from **tea-break Pilates:**

Neural arm exercise (page 84)

(c) Suggested exercise from **additional stretches:**

Shoulder stretch (page 86)

Carpal tunnel syndrome

- Move the wrist joint through its entire range of movement.

(a) Lift and lower fingers

(5–10 repetitions)

- Place the palm of the hand on a flat surface, spreading the fingers.
- Lift and lower fingers, one at a time.

(b) Wrist circles

(10 repetitions in each direction)

- Lift your arms to shoulder level in front of you, with elbows and wrists relaxed.

- Rotate your hands inwards at the wrists, towards your body.
- Then rotate the hands outwards, away from the body.

(c) Fists

(5–10 repetitions)

- Scrunch your fingers into fists, then open and extend the fingers.

(d) Walking fingers

(5–10 repetitions)

- Walk your fingers forwards and backwards along a flat surface.

(e) Wrist and finger shakes

- Lift your arms in front of you just below shoulder level, keeping the fingers and wrists relaxed.
- Shake your hands loosely from the wrists as if you are trying to dry them.

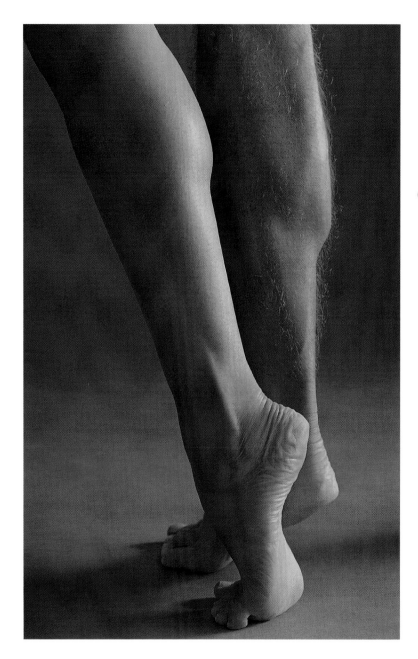

Note:

Avoid the following exercises:

- Press-ups – **step-by-step** section (page 68)
- Single and double leg kick – **more advanced** section (page 73 and 74).

8 Ankle and foot problems

It is imperative to correct postural alignment, with special emphasis on the hip, knee and foot alignment (*see* page 23).

Suggested exercises:

(a) Simple rises (*see* 'additional stretches', page 86).

(b) Ankle circles

(5–10 repetitions)

- Sit upright on a chair or exercise ball.
- Raise the right foot and circle it from the ankle outwards, away from the body.
- Repeat, circling inwards, towards the body.
- Repeat with the left foot.

(c) Lifting the arch

(10–20 repetitions)

- Sit upright on a chair or exercise ball, legs hip-width apart, knees bent, feet parallel.
- Lift the arches of the feet. Release the arches back to the starting position.

Note:

- Try to retain lengthened toes throughout.

(d) Spreading the toes

(10–20 repetitions)

- Sit on the mat, legs hip-width apart, knees bent.
- Fan and open your toes to spread them sideways. Relax back to the starting position.

7 Knee problems

Pilates exercises are excellent for knee strengthening, as they do not impose unnecessary stress on the knee. It is imperative to correct postural alignment, with special emphasis on the hip, knee and foot alignment, (*see* pages 23–24). All Pilates exercises that include knee flexion and extension are good. In a fully equipped Pilates studio, exercises on the Reformer are ideal for knee rehabilitation.

(a) Suggested exercise from the **warm-up** routine:

Repetitive marching on the spot (*see* page 46)

CONCLUSION

THE body is a wonderful machine but, like a great many machines, it has its weak areas and requires regular maintenance. It should be your goal to re-evaluate certain aspects of your lifestyle and to recognize the weak areas of your body. Only then are you in a position to work on the general maintenance of your body and strengthening the weak areas.

The shoulder joint and lower back are often especially vulnerable. The amount of time we spend sitting in front of television or computer screens and in vehicles subjects our bodies to high levels of stress. Fortunately, the abdominal strength that can be achieved through Pilates exercises will strengthen the vulnerable lower back. Correct shoulder placement and strengthening of the stabilizing muscles of the upper torso strengthens both the shoulder joint and upper body.

We have learned that well-aligned posture is the first step to redressing muscle imbalances in the body. The next step is exercise: its importance and value in preventing and treating physical and psychological diseases cannot be overemphasized.

Empower yourself with knowledge about your body. Understand which movements are or are not compatible with your joints, then strengthen your muscles through exercise, working to correct and improve your posture.

Through the Pilates programme of exercise, you can achieve your personal goals and reap the benefits.

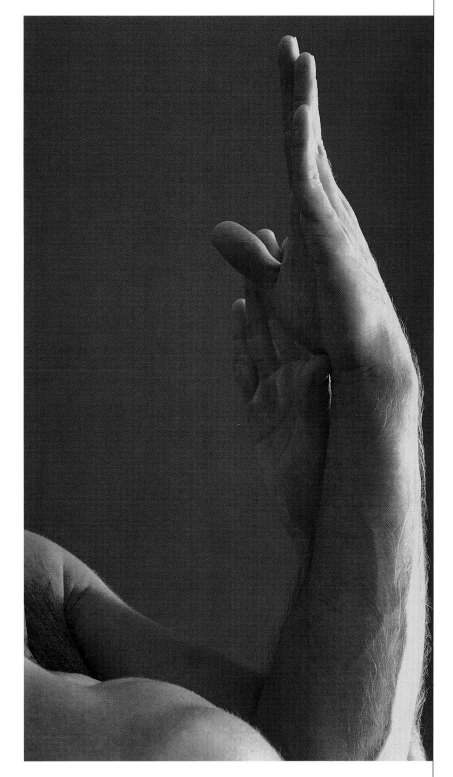

GLOSSARY

Abduction movement away from the midline of the trunk

Adduction movement towards the midline of the trunk

Agonist muscles most involved in an action

Antagonist muscles that work in co-operation with agonist muscles

Anterior in front

Anterior pelvic tilt forward tilt of pelvis

Belly to spine breathing pulling the navel towards the spine on exhalation

Cervical spine vertebrae of the neck (7 cervical vertebrae)

Contra-lateral relating to the opposite side

Cranio-vertebral flexion flexion of head on neck

Depression inferior movement of the shoulder girdle (returning to normal position from shoulder shrugging, pulling the shoulders down)

Dorsi-flexion bending movement of the ankle resulting in the top of the foot moving towards the shin

Elevation lifting the shoulder girdle (shrugging shoulders)

Eversion turning the sole of the foot outward

Expiration breathing out/exhalation

Extension straightening movement

External rotation turning movement away from the midline of the body

Flexed/flexion bending movement

Hyper-extend over-extension, where elbows or knees lock

Imprinted spine when the pelvis is tilted slightly so that the vertebrae of the lumbar spine (lower back) are imprinted into the mat

Internal rotation turning movement towards the midline of the body

Kyphosis an increased concavity of the thoracic curve of the spine

Lateral to the side

Lateral flexion side bending away from midline

Lordosis increased concavity of the lumbar curve of the spine (hollow back)

Lumbar lower back (five lumbar vertebrae)

Medial relating to the middle or centre

Neutral pelvis/spine the tips of the hip bones and pubic bone lie on the same plane

'Nod' position of the head as in cranio-vertebral flexion

Plumbline line running through the body, dissecting it in half, through the centre of the ear, shoulder, hip, knee and ankle (as illustrated in figure A on page 29)

Preparatory exercises easy exercises to be performed in place of the main exercise by those with physical problems, or by beginners until they build muscle strength

Posterior behind

Posterior pelvic tilt backward tilt of the pelvis

Powerhouse the 'centre' of the body between the hips and the ribs at the front and back of the torso

Prone position lying on the stomach

Protraction forward movement of shoulder girdle away from spine

Retraction backward movement of the shoulder girdle towards the spine

Rotation turning

Scoliosis sideward curvature of the spine

Supine lying on the back

Thoracic mid-spine (12 vertebrae)

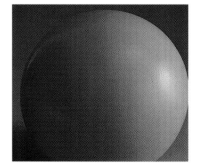

CONTACTS

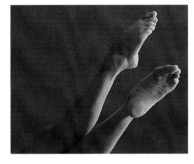

ASIA

Pilates Bodyworks
55 Market Street
Suite 03-01 Sinsov Building
Singapore 048941
Tel: +65 538 8922
Fax: +65 538 8622
E-mail: info@pilates.com.sg
Website: www.pilates.com.sg

AUSTRALIA

Body Arts & Science International
c/o International Pilates Training
Centre
Suite 41-42, Level 4
61 Marlborough St
Surrey Hills, Sydney NSW 2050
Tel: +61 (2) 9699 5509
Fax: +61 (2) 9698 0087
E-mail: pilatesint@bigpond.com

BAHAMAS

Pilates Academy
c/o Newbight General Delivery
Cat Island
Bahamas
Tel: +1242 342 7067
Website:
www.pilatesinternational.co.uk

CANADA

Canadian Pilates Association
PO Box 53559
984 West Broadway
Vancouver, British Columbia
V5Z-1K0
Website:
www.canadianpilatesassoc.com

Stott Pilates, Inc.
2200 Yonge St, Suite 1402
Toronto, Ontario M4S 2C6
Tel: +1 (416) 482 4050
Fax: +1 (416) 482 2742
E-mail: stott@stottpilates.com
Website: www.stottpilates.com

V.I. Pilates Fitness & Rehabilitation
579 Bay St
Victoria BC, VP5 Canada
Tel: +1 (250) 384 8686
E-mail: cvb@vipilates.ca

DENMARK

Copenhagen Pilates Studio
Longangstraede 37 B
1468 Copenhagen K
Tel: +45 3311 0088
E-mail: info@pilates-studio.dk
Website: www.pilates-studio.dk

FRANCE

Studio Pilates de Paris
39 rue du Temple
75006, Paris
Tel: +33 (1) 4272 9174
Fax: +33 (1) 4272 9187
E-mail: sebastien@obtpilates.com
Website: www.obtpilates.com

HOLLAND

The Pilates Studio Certification
Center, Netherlands
Keizerstraat 32
Den Haag, 2584 BJ
Tel: +31 (70) 350 8684
Fax: +31 (70) 322 8285
E-mail: info@pilates.nl
Website: www.pilates.nl

ITALY

Studio Pilates di Anna Maria Cova
Via Petrella 21
Milan 20124
Tel/Fax: +39 (02) 2951 0482
E-mail: info@pilatesineurope.it
Website: www.pilatesineurope.it

NEW ZEALAND

Level One, Willis Street Village,
142 Willis Street, Wellington
Tel: +64 (4) 384 1034
Fax: +64 (4) 384 1036
E-mail: pilates@nzsites.com
Website: www.nzsites.com/Pilates

Pilates Unlimited
18 Northcroft Street
Takapuna, Auckland
Tel/fax: +64 (9) 486 1018
E-mail: pilates@paradise.net.nz

NORWAY

Pilates Body Control, Oslo, Norway
Ropernveien 6A
1367 Snaroya
Tel: +47 6753 1536 / +47 9515 7253
Fax: +47 6753 1536
E-mail: greengeorgie@hotmail.com

Contacts

SOUTH AFRICA

P.L. Pilates
106 Campground Road
Rondebosch, Cape Town
Tel: +27 (21) 686 3153
E-mail: patl@netactive.co.za

Body Arts & Science International
c/o The Pilates Centre
86 Second St, Parkmoore
Sandton, Johannesburg
Tel: +27 (11) 784 3988

SPAIN

Estudio El Arte del Control
Calle Castanyer, 23
08022 Barcelona
E-mail: info@artecontrol-pilates.com
Website: www.artecontrol-pilates.com

SWEDEN

Body Control Studio
Atlasgatan 12
11320 Stockholm
Tel/fax: +946 (478) 345 347
Website: www.pilates.stockholm.nu

SWITZERLAND

Pilates Exercise
Nordstrasse 145
CH-8037 Zürich
Tel: +41 (1) 350 2277
Fax: +41 (1) 350 2278
E-mail: box@pilates-exercise.ch
Website: www.pilates.ch

UK

Body Control Pilates Association
14 Neal's Yard, Covent Garden
London, WC2H 9DP
Tel: +44 (207) 379 3734
Fax: +44 (207) 379 7551
E-mail: info@bodycontrol.co.uk
Website: www.bodycontrol.co.uk

Pilates Foundation UK Ltd
80 Camden Rd
London, E17 7NF
Tel: +44 (171) 781 859
E-mail: admin@pilatesfoundation.com
Website: www.pilatesfoundation.com

Pilates International
Unit 1, Broadbent Close
20/22 Highgate High Street
London N6 5JG
Tel/fax: +44 020 83481442
E-mail:
pilates@pilatesinternational.co.uk
Website:
www.pilatesinternational.co.uk

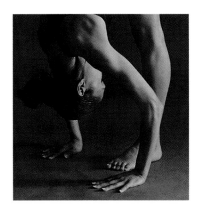

USA

Pilates Method Alliance
PO Box 370906
Miami, FL 33137 0906
Toll free: 866 573 4945
Tel: +1 (305) 573 4946
Fax: +1 (305) 573 4461
E-mail:
info@pilatesmethodalliance.org
Website:
www.pilatesmethodalliance.org

The Pilates & Physical Theory Center
of Seattle
413 Fairview Avenue North
Seattle, WA 98109
Tel: +1 (206) 405 3560
Fax: +1 (206) 405 3938
E-mail:
customercare@pilatesseattle.com
Website: www.pilatesseattle.com

Performing Arts Physical Therapy &
The Pilates Studio ® of Los Angeles
8704 Santa Monica Blvd, Suite 300
West Hollywood, CA 90069
Tel: +1 (310) 659 1077
Fax: +1 (310) 659 1163
E-mail: info@pilatestherapy.com
Website: www.pilatestherapy.com

Energy Balancing Pilates Studio
The Harmony Group
10 Grand Avenue
Englewood, NJ 07631
Tel: +1 (201) 871 4415
Fax: +1 (201) 913 7937
E-mail: kristi@theharmonygroup.com
Website: www.theharmonygroup.com

INDEX

ACKNOWLEDGEMENTS

I would like to thank dance colleague, Tracy Dawber, for introducing me to Pilates; all my Pilates students for their valuable input; as well as physiotherapist and Pilates practitioner, Vivienne Schulze, for reading the manuscript and making suggestions. Grateful thanks are also due to commissioning editor, Karyn Richards, for her enthusiasm; models Mandy Stober, Linda Smit, Antonie Nel and Hanri Loots for their willingness and time; and my brother-in-law, Royston Lamond, for his interest, encouragement and artistic input. I would also like to thank my son, Michael, for his patient help with the computer; and my husband, Peter, and son, Jon Craig, for their love and support.

PHOTOGRAPHIC CREDITS

All photographs by Ryno Reyneke, except:

p11: Photo Access

p12: Photo Access

p13, p14 top: Pine Mountain Productions (IC Rapoport)

p15 middle, bottom: Merrithew Corp*

p25: Gallo Images

p26: J&B Photographers (BarrieWilkins)

p27: Sporting Pictures (UK) Ltd

*For more information on Stott Pilates equipment, training and videos, tel: +1 (416) 482 4050; www.stottpilates.com